BASIC FACT
FRACTU

PATRICK S.H. BROWNE
MA, BM, BCh, FRCS
Reader in Orthopaedics
University of Tasmania

SECOND EDITION

Blackwell Scientific Publications

OXFORD LONDON EDINBURGH

BOSTON PALO ALTO MELBOURNE

© 1983, 1988 by
Blackwell Scientific Publications
Editorial offices:
Osney Mead, Oxford OX2 0EL
  (*Orders*: Tel. 0865−240201)
8 John Street, London WC1N 2ES
23 Ainslie Place, Edinburgh EH3
  6AJ
Three Cambridge Center, Suite 208,
  Cambridge, MA 02142, USA
667 Lytton Avenue, Palo Alto
  California 94301, USA
107 Barry Street, Carlton
  Victoria 3053, Australia

First published 1983
Second edition 1988

Set by Setrite Typesetters Ltd
Hong Kong
Printed and bound
in Great Britain

DISTRIBUTORS

USA
  Year Book Medical Publishers
  200 North LaSalle Street
  Chicago, Illinois 60601
  (*Orders*: Tel. 312−726−9733)

Canada
  The C.V. Mosby Company
  5240 Finch Avenue East
  Scarborough, Ontario
  (*Orders*: Tel. 416−298−1588)

Australia
  Blackwell Scientific Publications
  (Australia) Pty Ltd
  107 Barry Street
  Carlton, Victoria 3053
  (*Orders*: Tel. (03) 347−0300)

British Library
Cataloguing in Publication Data
Browne, Patrick S.H.
  Basic facts of fractures. — 2nd
ed.
  1. Fractures
  I. Title
  617'.15   RD101

ISBN 0−632−02128−4

Contents

Preface

TO FIRST EDITION

The basic facts of fractures and of their management are described in this book. There are no details of operative treatment or of manipulations (beyond those for Colles' fracture and dislocation of the shoulder). These procedures are best performed in hospital and the learning of them best obtained by example.

I have used a 'system of stars' to indicate difficulties in the management of particular fractures. This system was used by Professor George Perkins in his book *Fractures and Dislocations*; my indications are slightly different from his:

* These fractures can be managed by simple treatment and will unite without complications. They can be managed quite adequately by any doctor at his office with the minimum of equipment.

** These fractures require hospital treatment and may require manipulation under a general anaesthetic. They can usually be managed by a junior doctor in training with indirect supervision.

*** These fractures require specialist management. They should not be treated by junior doctors without direct supervision.

**** These fractures frequently lead to bad results no matter who manages them. They should not, under any circumstances, be treated by junior doctors.

I thank all those who helped me with this book, in particular, I thank Mrs. Hilary Goldsmid for the excellence of her illustrations.

TO SECOND EDITION

The second edition of this book includes a revision both of text and illustrations. It was necessary to do this as there have been many advances and innovations in treatment of fractures over the past five years.

The chapter on knee injuries has been rewritten, otherwise the general form remains the same.

common fractures — pediatric forearm 1st
— elderly wrist 2nd
— " hip 3rd

1 General Principles

Bone is composed of an organic matrix known as osteoid. This consists of collagen fibres embedded in a cementing gel of protein polysaccharide. A mineral known as apatite consisting of calcium and phosphate is deposited on the collagen fibres as needle shaped crystals.

The collagen fibres in adult bone are aligned to parallel the average compression and tension stresses to which the bone is subject. The apatite crystals are similarly orientated on the collagen fibres.

Bone strength is dependent on the normal formation of osteoid and mineral. It is dependent on this alignment parallel to the average stresses to which the bone is subject.

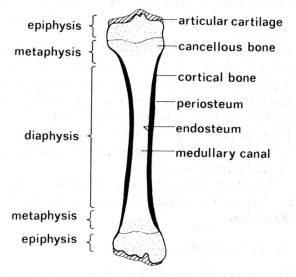

epiphysis — articular cartilage

metaphysis — cancellous bone

— cortical bone

— periosteum

diaphysis — endosteum

— medullary canal

metaphysis

epiphysis

Fig. 1.1. Parts of bone

In adults long bones consist of tubes of cortical bone. The hollow centre contains marrow, and the occasional trabeculae of cancellous bone (Fig. 1.1). The ends of bone are

1

expanded towards the articular surface. This expansion is the metaphysis — here the cortex is thinned but arcades of cancellous bone supporting the articular surface are more pronounced. These arcades also parallel the average stress to which the ends of the bone is subject and are aligned to transmit these stresses to the diaphysis (Fig. 1.2).

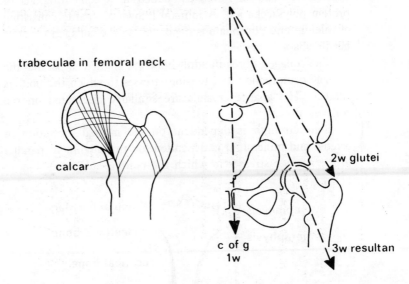

Fig. 1.2. Trabeculae aligned along lines of stress, w = body weight

The shaft of a long bone is ensheathed in a layer of periosteum. The outer portion of this layer is fibrous tissue — the inner portion (cambium) contains primitive mesenchymal cells.

The lining of the marrow cavity is known as endosteum and is also the source of primitive mesenchymal cells. Pluripotent mesenchymal cells are present in the periosteum, endosteum and also the trabeculae. They can develop into (a) osteoblasts which lay down new bone, or (b) osteoclasts which absorb bone.

This activity is stimulated by trauma (fracture), by infection or by tumours which tend to displace the periosteum. Such lesions cause a periosteal reaction which is visible on X-rays as new bone.

The cortex of a long bone is made of well-organised compact bone (Fig. 1.3). This bone is organised in a series of Haversian systems (each of which is an osteon) based on a central blood vessel. Osteocytes are embedded in the bone surrounding the blood vessel and are joined to it by minute canaliculi. The osteocytes maintain bone and are associated with its biochemical turnover. The alignment of the lamellae of each osteon is slightly different from its neighbour. This varied alignment adds strength to the bone particularly as regards tangential stresses.

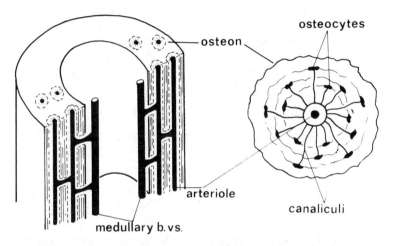

Fig. 1.3. Haversian system

Bone is less able to withstand torsional stresses than tangential stresses. It is easier to fracture a bone by twisting it. Torsional stresses produce a spiral fracture (see Fig. 1.7). These fractures are usually 'low energy' fractures and are associated with a lesser degree of soft tissue and skin damage.

Tangential stresses produce a transverse or short oblique fracture. More severe violence results in a comminuted fracture with a butterfly fragment (see Fig. 1.7). This type of fracture is usually a 'high energy' fracture and is associated with a greater degree of soft tissue and skin damage.

Cancellous bone is present towards the ends of long bones. The trabeculae are arranged adjacent to blood vessels — they are thinner and less complex than the lamellae of the cortex.

3

The trabeculae are arranged to parallel the average compression and tension stresses to which the ends of bone are subject.

When a fracture occurs through cancellous bone it is associated with some crushing of the trabeculae. The blood supply of the trabeculae is good and cancellous bone heals rapidly. However, there is usually some residual deformity due to crushing of the trabeculae. Vertebral bodies consist of cancellous bone and may sustain a crush fracture; as a result they become wedge-shaped (Fig. 1.4).

normal body

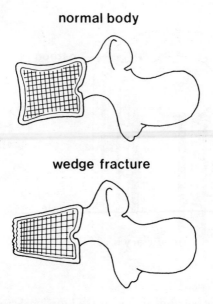

wedge fracture

Fig. 1.4. Wedge fracture

Any lesion which interferes with the normal arrangement of cortical or cancellous bone tends to weaken it. An example of such a lesion is Paget's disease. In this condition there is no deficiency in the amount of bone. However, the internal architecture of the bone is disorganised and weakened. Long bones become bowed and liable to pathological fractures.

In all people, there is a continuous turnover of bone — this process is known as remodelling. It is much more active and more rapid in children. Each individual osteon can be removed by osteoclasts and replaced by osteoblasts. This replacement can occur in a slightly different location in response to altered stresses. In old people, and in areas relieved of usual stresses, this replacement process lags behind the remodelling process and osteoporosis results. This process of remodelling:

1 Permits a micro repair mechanism for wear and tear of minor trauma. It acts as a built-in protection against 'fatigue' (in the metallurgical sense).

2 Permits realignment of lamellae in response to change of loads.

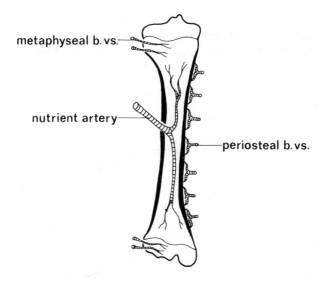

Fig. 1.5. Blood supply of a long bone

The blood supply of an adult bone is from (Fig. 1.5):

1 A central nutrient artery which supplies the marrow endosteum and the inner two-thirds of the cortex of the diaphysis;

2 Vessels from the periosteum which supply the outer one third of the cortex;

3 Various vessels in the metaphyseal region.

Lesions which affect the blood supply to a bone causes that portion supplied to die. A fracture causes interruption of the blood supply of cortical bone. There is necessarily some dead bone at the fracture site. The amount of dead bone depends on the shape of the fracture and on the severity of the original deforming force. Cancellous bone has a good blood supply, there is only a small amount of dead bone at the fracture site and delayed union is not usually a problem.

PATHOLOGICAL FRACTURES

A pathological fracture occurs through an area of previously diseased bone. It may occur spontaneously if the bone is sufficiently eroded. The causes of pathological fractures can be listed:
1 Generalised bone disease such as:
  osteoporosis
  osteogenesis imperfecta
  Paget's disease
2 Tumours — secondary deposits:
  most commonly the breast in females
  most commonly the lung in males
  malignant myeloma
3 Bone cysts and fibrous dysplasia
4 Other conditions:
  chronic osteomyelitis
  radio necrosis
  avascular necrosis

STRESS FRACTURES

A stress (or fatigue) fracture of bone is found in an area subjected to excessive persistent stress. Initially they are difficult to diagnose as X-rays show only a minute crack. Repeat films after a few weeks reveal a cloud of callus at the fracture site (Fig. 1.6).

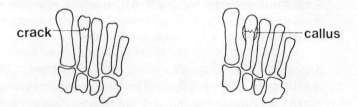

crack — — callus

Fig. 1.6. Stress fracture in the neck of the second metatarsal

The commonest site for a stress fracture is in the neck of the second metatarsal. It may cause severe foot pain. This fracture is known as a 'March fracture' as it is frequently seen in army recruits after a long route march. Stress fractures are also seen in the tibia or fibula in athletes and in professional dancers.

A bone scan is the most sensitive method of diagnosing stress fractures. As a result of its use the incidence of stress fractures has been shown to be much more frequent than previously supposed. Many cases of 'shin splints' and other painful conditions in athletes have been demonstrated as being due to a stress fracture. The treatment is rest.

TYPES OF FRACTURE

A compound fracture

A compound fracture is a fracture associated with an open wound. Unless properly treated the fracture site is liable to become infected. Two types are described:

1 Compound from within — the bone fragments themselves pierce the skin;

2 Compound from without — the skin is disrupted from without and the bone then fractured. This type of fracture is more likely to become infected.

A complicated fracture

A complicated fracture is associated with damage to other vital structures such as nerves, arteries or viscera.

A comminuted fracture (Fig. 1.7)

A comminuted fracture has more than two main fragments. Such a fracture may be produced by severe violence or by crushing with considerable soft tissue damage. However, it also can occur in bones which are simply weakened by osteoporosis.

A crush fracture (Fig. 1.4)

A crush fracture occurs in cancellous bone and involves crushing of the trabeculae. Such fractures are common in the vertebral bodies producing wedging.

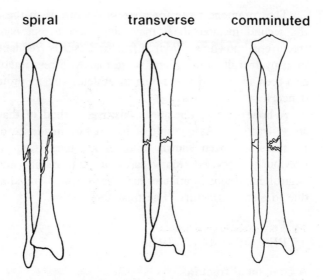

spiral   transverse   comminuted

Fig. 1.7. Three different types of long bone fracture

Fractures involving a joint
These are often very painful as they are accompanied by a
a haemarthrosis. As the joint surfaces are damaged, joint stiffness follows and may be very resistant to treatment. In later
years degenerative changes may occur in the joint. These joints
may become painful, particularly if they are weight-bearing
joints.

Some joint fractures are associated with ligament damage.
Unless the ligaments are allowed to repair themselves, joint
instability can result.

An osteochondral fracture (Fig. 1.8)
An osteochondral fragment may be sheared off the articular
surface. It consists of a thin layer of bone attached to articular
cartilage. If allowed to remain free it can form a loose body.
This may cause symptoms of locking.

A chondral fracture
A chondral fracture contains only cartilage. Otherwise it is
similar to an osteochondral fracture. It is not visible on X-ray.
These fractures may be associated with other knee joint injuries.

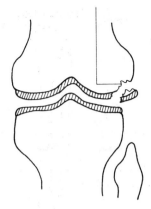

Fig. 1.8. Osteochondral fracture

An avulsion fracture (Fig. 1.9)

An avulsion fracture occurs when the bony attachment of a tendon or ligament is torn away. They can occur from excessive muscle violence. The bony fragments are often widely separated because of muscle contraction. Avulsion fractures often require open reduction and internal fixation to restore normal function.

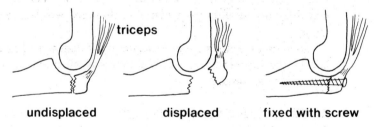

undisplaced   displaced   fixed with screw

Fig. 1.9. An avulsion fracture

A greenstick fracture (Fig. 1.10)

A greenstick fracture occurs in children. Childrens' bones are less brittle than adults. They have a thicker periosteum. A greenstick fracture consists of an impaction or buckling of one cortex and separation of the cortex opposite to the deforming

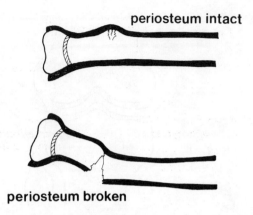

periosteum intact

periosteum broken

Fig. 1.10. Buckle and greenstick fracture

force. Reduction of these fractures can be obtained by reversing the deforming force. This reduction can easily be maintained in plaster as the periosteum on one side is strong and intact.

A buckle (wrinkle or torus) fracture is an undisplaced greenstick fracture. The periosteum is probably intact over both cortices (Fig. 1.10).

Fractures near the growth plate
Fractures in children frequently involve this area. Damage to the growth plate may result in growth arrest. This is usually partial but may be complete.

A complete growth arrest will result in shortening of the limb. The younger the child, the shorter the limb will be in adult life. Partial damage to the growth plate will result in deformities. The growth will be stopped on one side of the epiphysis and will continue on the other; as the child grows so the deformity will become more and more severe.

Salter and Harris classified fractures about the growth plate (Fig. 1.11):
Type I: Separation of the growth plate and epiphysis from the metaphysis. This may be difficult to see on X-ray.
Type II: The fracture line separates the growth plate from the metaphysis but includes a triangular portion of the metaphysis. This is the commonest type of fracture.

metaphysis

growth
plate

epiphysis

1. separation of growth
plate & epiphysis

2. 1+flake of metaphysis

3. portion of growth
plate & epiphysis

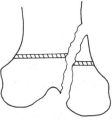

4. portion of metaphysis,
growth plate & epiphysis

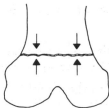

5. crushing of growth plate

Fig. 1.11. Growth plate fractures

Type III: An intra-articular fracture involves the separation of a portion of the epiphysis and growth plate.

Type IV: A vertical fracture through the epiphysis, growth plate and metaphysis — if displaced this requires accurate reduction. If it is not accurately reduced then growth arrest will involve a portion of the growth plate.

Type V: A crushing injury of the growth plate. This lesion

11

has the worst prognosis for growth arrest and is difficult to diagnose as it is almost impossible to see on X-ray.

Types I and II have the best prognosis as regards growth arrest. Types IV and V have the worst prognosis.

LIGAMENT SPRAINS AND RUPTURES

If a joint is subjected to excessive violence its collateral ligaments are liable to damage.

Sprain

This occurs if the violence is not severe enough to cause a complete disruption. On careful, clinical examination no laxity

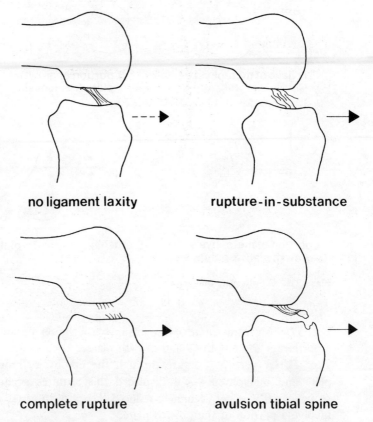

no ligament laxity   rupture-in-substance

complete rupture   avulsion tibial spine

Fig. 1.12. Rupture of anterior cruciate ligament

of the ligament can be detected. Immobilisation for two or three weeks will permit healing and recovery will eventually occur with no significant loss of function.

Ligament rupture
This occurs in a variety of ways (Fig. 1.12):

Rupture in the substance of the ligament. Individual ligament fibres are ruptured at varying levels. At operation the ligament appears contused and stretched — on clinical examination it is lax. This is the common type of ligament rupture.

Complete rupture of the ligament. This can occur either in the substance of the ligament or at its bony attachment.

Avulsion fracture. A small fragment of bone is pulled away at the site of ligament attachment. Such avulsion fractures will heal if they are accurately replaced. This may require an operation.

A joint dislocation occurs as a result of violence. The two articular surfaces are completely separated. There is necessarily severe ligament and capsule damage.

A subluxation is an incomplete dislocation.

NERVE INJURIES

Peripheral nerve lesions
Peripheral nerve injuries are classified by their severity (Fig. 1.13).

Neuropraxia
This is a benign disturbance of nerve function lasting only a short time (a few days). It is a physiological interruption of peripheral nerve function. The lesion is often incomplete with motor paralysis but some residual sensory function.

Axonotmesis
The nerve fibres are damaged sufficiently for the individual axons to degenerate. However the endoneural tubes remain intact so that complete recovery can occur. This type of lesion is common with fractures.

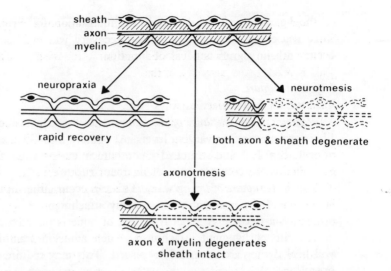

Fig. 1.13. Peripheral nerve injury

Neurotmesis
This indicates either actual anatomical division of the nerve or severe scarring such that spontaneous regeneration is impossible. Surgical repair is required. This type of lesion occurs with lacerations. It also occurs after severe traction injuries or ischaemia.

After section a nerve fibre undergoes *Wallerian degeneration*. This involves:
1 Degeneration of the axon;
2 The myelin sheath breaks up;
3 The endoneural tubes narrow;
4 In due course the muscle end/plates deteriorate and the muscle fibres atrophy. The sensory endings also become atrophied.
During the reparative process:
1 Debris is removed by macrophages;
2 Fibroblasts enter the gap and tend to form fibrous tissue. Also the Schwann cells of the endoneural tube proliferate and cross the gap and reform the endoneural tubes. If the gap is too large fibrous tissue predominates and it cannot be bridged by the proliferating Schwann cells;
3 Axon fibrils grow down the spaces between the Schwann

cells and traverse the lesion to enter the distal endoneural tube. They will eventually reach the end organs;
4 New myelin sheath is developed and nerve function returns. This process takes several months.

Acute peripheral nerve injuries
All patients suffering lacerations or fractures should be suspected of having nerve lesions. They should be examined to exclude them. Such examination should include testing the movements subserved by the relevant muscles. (This may be difficult in patients with painful injured limbs.) Sensation should be tested. (In recently injured patients, gross pin prick is probably the most useful.)

Any laceration which is likely to involve a nerve should be explored by a formal operation with torniquet and general anaesthesia. A laceration on the volar aspect of the wrist is best treated thus as either or both median and ulnar nerves can be damaged from such an injury.

Lesions associated with fractures are usually either a neuropraxia or axonotmesis. Such lesions will usually recover and do not require operation initially. If they do not recover then the lesion must be explored.

Brachial plexus lesions
These are usually traction injuries caused by forced lateral flexion of the head on the trunk. Such injuries occur most frequently in adults as a result of motorcycle accidents. They also occur as birth injuries. The traction injury can cause a neuropraxia, axonotmesis or neurotmesis or frequently a combination of these lesions in the different elements of the plexus. High speed motorcycle accidents can result in actual avulsion of the nerve roots from the cervical spinal cord (Fig. 1.14).

Birth trauma
This may be a benign lesion which recovers completely. The most common residual lesion is an Erb's palsy and the lesion is stated to occur at Erb's point, the junction of C5 and C6 nerve roots. These patients have a residual paresis of deltoid, of elbow flexors, of supinator and of wrist extensors.

A Klumpke's paralysis is less common and involves C8 and

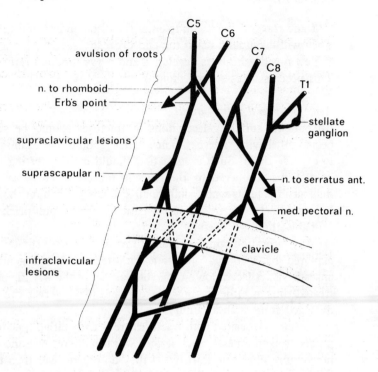

Fig. 1.14. Brachial plexus lesions

T1 nerve roots causing a paresis of finger flexors and the intrinsic muscles of the hand.

Infraclavicular lesions
These may be associated with a fractured clavicle or dislocated shoulder. The lesion is often incomplete involving cords and nerves and the prognosis for recovery is usually good.

Supraclavicular lesions
These patients frequently have a completely paralysed upper limb sparing only the rhomboids and serratus anterior. There may be complete sensory loss as well in which case the prognosis for recovery is poor. Recovery however may occur over a period of two years from injury and it is best not to be dogmatic in assessing these patients.

Avulsion of cervical nerve roots
These patients have an irrecoverable lesion proximal to the posterior root ganglion. They may have a Horner's syndrome (constricted pupil, ptosis and enophthalmos) due to avulsion of the ramus from T1 to the stellate ganglion.

A myelogram may show meningoceles along the affected cervical nerve roots. Avulsion of these nerve roots may rupture the dural sleeves related to them and permit the dye to leak.

Treatment
The treatment of brachial plexus lesions is essentially conservative. To date no attempts at repair have been demonstrated to show any worthwhile improvement of function.

In patients with birth, infraclavicular and supraclavicular lesions some recovery is possible for at least two years from injury. These patients should be subjected to persistent physiotherapy to preserve the mobility of joints. They should also be splinted to prevent deformities.

After two years reconstructive operations may be undertaken. If the shoulder is flail it is best arthrodesed. Various tendon transfer operations can be performed to make the best use of residual muscle function.

Patients who have avulsion of the nerve roots have no hope of recovery. The diagnosis is confirmed by a myelogram showing meningoceles. These patients are probably best treated by providing them with a specially designed lightweight brachial plexus splint. On occasion the limb has been so painful that amputation is advised.

surgical fusion of joint

FRACTURE HEALING

The process of fracture healing is different for cortical and for cancellous bone. The process is altered by internal fixation.

Healing of cortical bone (Fig. 1.15)
1 As a result of fracture, bleeding occurs from the damaged bone ends and damaged soft tissues. The blood clots. Osteocytes imprisoned in their lacunae near the fracture site lose their blood supply — a certain amount of bone dies.
2 Capillaries, from the periosteum and endosteum invade the

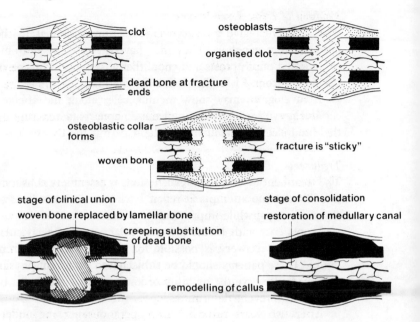

Fig. 1.15. Bone healing

clot and gradually transform it to granulation tissue. Osteoblasts, probably derived from the periosteum and endosteum, proliferate into the granulation tissue.

3 This cellular reaction raises the periosteum away from the bone cortex and an osteoblastic collar is formed. This produces primitive woven bone. In time the woven bone proliferation reaches across the fracture gap. The fracture becomes more stable although still mobile. This stage is reached about three weeks after fracture — the fracture is 'sticky'.

4 Over the succeeding weeks the collar of woven bone becomes more dense and is gradually transformed to lamellar bone. When there is no detectable movement — the fracture is 'clinically united'.

5 After union remodelling occurs. Excess callus is removed and the medullary cavity reformed. When the process is advanced the fracture is said to be 'consolidated'.

In normal adults a cortical bone takes about three months to unite.

Healing of cancellous bone

The osteocytes in the trabeculae have a more profuse blood supply.

There is little callus formed. Bone union occurs fairly rapidly as the gap is bridged directly. This only occurs in areas of direct contact.

Healing of fractures in cancellous bone is necessarily associated with some degree of collapse.

Such fractures will unite in about six weeks.

Healing of fractures after open reduction and internal fixation

At operation the clot is removed from between the fracture ends. The early osteoblastic collar is disturbed and sometimes removed. The usual biological processes of fracture healing are disturbed and bone union is delayed. The fixation device must be adequate to compensate for this delayed bone union. The effects of internal fixation are listed below.

1 Non-rigid fixation — union depends on the eventual formation of woven bone derived from both periosteum and endosteum.

2 Intramedullary fixation — union depends on woven bone from the periosteum (Fig. 1.16).

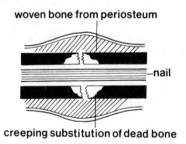

woven bone from periosteum

—nail

creeping substitution of dead bone

Fig. 1.16. Intramedullary fixation

3 Rigid compression plating — no periosteal callus is seen. Union must depend on endosteal revascularisation of the area of dead bone. A process is described of direct osteoblastic proliferation from lamellar bone — similar to Haversian canal remodelling. This process takes some months in adult patients,

and depends on how much dead bone is present at the fracture site (Fig. 1.17).

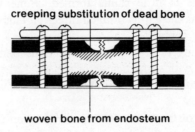

Fig. 1.17. Compression plating

Fractures with internal fixation can be reduced anatomically and often mobilised early.

However, the implant must be strong enough and durable enough to support the fracture for some months. The surgeon using it must be skilled in its applications.

Childrens' fractures

Childrens' fractures unite much more easily and rapidly. Remodelling is a more complete process. An incomplete reduction is often acceptable. Only rotational deformities are not well corrected.

Delayed union

Factors which interfere with fracture union include:

1 Local factors:
   blood supply of bone
   infection
   a wide gap between bone ends with interposition
      of extraneous tissue
2 General factors:
   poor nutrition
   Vitamin C deficiency
   old age

Delayed union is said to occur when a fracture does not unite within an expected time. It may unite eventually given persistent immobilisation. An uncomplicated fracture of the tibial shaft in adults would be expected to unite in thirteen weeks. If it had not united in eighteen weeks it would be classified as delayed union and considered for bone grafting. Delayed union is a diagnosis which depends on:

1 Clinical signs:
  mobility
  pain and tenderness at fracture site
2 X-ray:
  shows incomplete callus with the fracture gap still
    detectable

Non-union

Non-union is a later stage. Such a fracture will never unite without bone grafting.

Clinical signs — obvious mobility;

X-rays — show sclerosed bone with the ends rounded off and a large gap between the bone ends.

Malunion

Malunion is defined as union of a fracture with an unacceptable deformity.

BONE GRAFTING

The usual treatment of delayed union and non-union of fractures is bone grafting. Bone grafts are obtained from various sources:

1 *Autogenous* grafts taken from the patient himself. There are no problems of immune reactions or of sterilisation. Some cells from autogenous grafts may survive at the recipient site. Types of autogenous grafts include:
  strips or chips of cancellous bone from the iliac crest
  blocks of cortical bone from the tibia
  whole bone from the fibula
2 *Homogenous* grafts of cadaveric bone. These must be freeze dried and specially sterilised. The bone cells are dead.
3 *Heterogenous* deproteinised bone (from other species).
  The function of bone grafts:
1 Some bone cells from autogenous cancellous bone grafts survive at the recipient site.
2 Bone grafts induce osteogenesis. This is accomplished by

stimulating osteoblasts to form bone and stimulating the formation of osteoblasts from primitive mesenchymal cells.

Cancellous grafts from the iliac crest have the greatest osteogenic inductive capacity. Heterogenous deproteinised grafts have practically none.

3 The dead graft acts as a scaffold to which woven bone becomes attached. Later it is completely vascularised and replaced by lamellar bone.

4 Block grafts (as from the tibia) have a structural function. The Phemister procedure is the most common operation used for bone grafting. The fracture is exposed and strips of cancellous bone from the iliac crest are laid on the surface beneath the periosteum.

Living bone transplants can be used for certain procedures. A block of iliac crest or a portion of fibula is developed on a vascular pedicle. The pedicle can be anastomosed to vessels at the recipient site. The living bone is incorporated directly.

COMPLICATIONS OF FRACTURES

The complications of fractures can be classified as follows:

Immediate complications — within days of fracture
Delayed complications — within weeks or months of fracture
Late complications — years after fracture

Immediate complications
These depend on the anatomy of the fracture and certain fractures are particularly liable to certain immediate complications. Examination of a patient with a fracture must include examination for these complications.

Injury to nerves
The nerve lesion is usually either a neuropraxia or axonotmesis. Recovery is usual in due course after reduction of the fracture. A nerve lesion is not necessarily an indication to explore a fracture surgically.

Injury to arteries (Fig. 1.18)
At time of fracture:
transection of artery

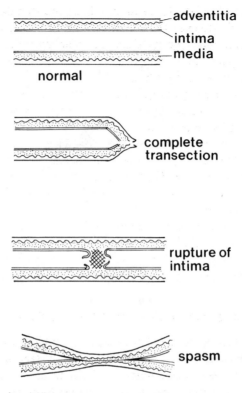

Fig. 1.18. Arterial injuries

contusion of artery (with endothelial rupture and thrombosis)
arterial spasm
Some hours after fracture:
'closed compartment syndrome' (Fig. 1.19)
Involvement of a major artery is usually an indication to explore the fracture surgically. An arterial contusion is the commonest cause of arterial occlusion immediately following a fracture. The damaged segment should be resected and if possible repaired by a vein graft.
The deep fascia divides the constituents of a limb into several compartments. A fracture of the shaft of a limb bone is associated with damage to muscle and bleeding into these compartments. If the fascia is undamaged, the pressure in the

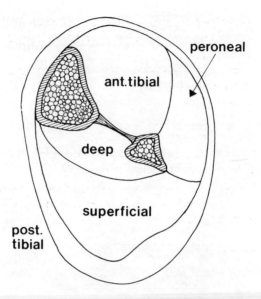

Fig. 1.19. Fascial compartments of lower leg

closed compartment rises and eventually the blood supply to the muscles is jeopardised. The limb is excessively painful and swollen and other signs of arterial insufficiency are present; such as pallor, paresis, paraesthesiae and decreased temperature. If unrelieved the muscle dies and is eventually replaced by fibrous tissues — a contracture results (such as Volkmann's contracture). Many such cases were at one time ascribed to too tight plasters and dressings. This is still a possibility.

The treatment of a patient with a closed compartment syndrome involves:

release of plaster and dressings down to the skin;

the operation of fasciotomy to relieve the closed compartment.

The signs and symptoms of vascular insufficiency must be remembered. When present they require immediate action for their relief:

the patient will complain of pain,

the pain is persistent and may get worse,

the pain is more severe on passive movement,

6 P's

there may be loss of active movements,
colour changes — duskiness and eventually a mottled pallor,
swelling,
sensory changes — tingling and numbness,
decreased temperature,
absent pulses.

Injuries to viscera

Fractures of the pelvis, spine and lower ribs may be associated with lesions of the abdominal viscera.

Fractures of the ribs are so frequently associated with lesions of the lung and pleura that they are properly cared for by thoracic surgeons.

Injuries to the skin

Compound fractures.

Injuries to the joints

Such injuries are often associated with a painful haemarthrosis. They can be classified as follows:

Osteochondral or chondral fractures — these tend not to heal and persist as loose bodies causing the symptoms of locking or instability;

Per-articular fractures which transgress the articular surface. These tend to be followed by joint stiffness and later degenerative changes;

Fracture dislocations — these are often unstable and difficult to hold reduced. They often require open reduction and internal fixation.

Complications of severe trauma

Patients with multiple injuries or with severe lower limb fractures are liable to develop other complications associated with hypovolaemic shock.

Shock

This clinical entity occurs after trauma. The patient becomes pale and cold and has a rapid pulse — he is relatively immobile. There are two main components to shock:

Neurogenic shock — probably due to the rapid influx of sensory impulses occurring on injury. This component responds rapidly to recumbency and splinting of the injured part and reassurance.

Hypovolaemic shock — this is due to actual loss of circulating blood volume associated with injury. Its severity depends on the rate and the amount of blood loss. In most patients blood loss is a continuing process until definitive treatment can be instituted. A patient in hypovolaemic shock requires immediate restoration of his blood volume.

Shock lung syndrome (post traumatic anoxia)
A patient with a significant large bone fracture or suffering from multiple injuries is liable to develop acute pulmonary complications.

These are characterised by increasing dysponea and respiratory embarrassment and a lowered arterial oxygen content. At post-mortem the lungs are found to be oedematous with local areas of collapse. Various factors have been considered to be responsible for this:
1 Actual lung damage from initial injury,
2 Embolism from damaged tissues — including fat emboli,
3 Over-transfusion in treating hypovolaemic shock,
4 Oedema may be secondary to water and electrolyte retention in response to injury.

Patients with this syndrome are severely ill and the mortality is high. Treatment is with positive pressure ventilation.

Fat embolism syndrome
This syndrome is similar to the shock lung syndrome. The patients become disorientated a few hours after injury. They become dyspnoeic and have a raised pulse rate. Patients severely affected show petechiae and have a typical appearance on chest X-ray. The arterial oxygen content is low.

In definite cases the serum lipase is raised and fat globules can be demonstrated in the urine.

These patients may become severely ill. They are best treated with positive pressure ventilation with high oxygen concentration until the condition resolves itself.

26

Delayed complications

Infection
After compound fractures — see p. 44;
After operations on fractures.
Secondary osteomyelitis can follow compound fractures or operations on fractures. It is very resistant to treatment once established and is associated with avascular bone and non-union. The presence of foreign material such as fixation devices tends to potentiate the infection.

Joint stiffness
This is a complication of all fractures particularly those treated by plaster immobilisation. The patient should be seen to move all joints which are mobile. This requires supervision.

Intra-articular fractures are particularly prone to joint stiffness. Fractures of the neck of the humerus are also particularly prone to joint stiffness.

Malunion
This occurs when a fracture has united in an unacceptable position. It may require an osteotomy to correct it.

For *delayed union* and *non-union* see pp. 20–1.

Late complications

Shortening
This is only a real problem after fractures of the lower limb. It can cause a limp and some degree of pelvic tilt. The latter is responsible for back ache. In brief:
Shortening of less than one centimetre is rarely noticed by the patient;
Shortening of less than four centimetres is readily compensated by a shoe raise;
Shortening over four centimetres is disabling and the compensatory shoe raise is clumsy and noticeable.

Residual deformity
This results from malunion. Rotational deformity often escapes the notice of the treating surgeon until too late. Remodelling of rotational deformities is poor.

Chapter 1

Osteoarthritis
This occurs in a damaged joint. If the joint is weight bearing it may cause disabling symptoms.

Osteoarthritis also occurs in a malaligned joint, secondary to malunion of shaft fractures.

Avascular necrosis
When a large portion of bone loses its blood supply, it dies and undergoes changes of avascular necrosis. It appears sclerotic on X-ray and collapses down and causes severe pain. Areas particularly affected are:

Head of the femur after displaced sub-capital fractures;
Body of the talus after a fracture dislocation or complete dislocation.
Proximal pole of the scaphoid after fracture of the waist.

Growth plate damage
This occurs in children after fractures adjacent to the growth plate. It can cause shortening of a limb or gross deformities (see p. 10).

2 Management of Fractures

FIRST AID

1 Ensure clear airway.
2 Restore circulating blood volume to combat shock.
3 Splintage of fractures:
   Upper arm and shoulder lesions — a sling and bind arm to the side
   Forearm and hand — splint and sling
   Lesions of thigh and knee — Thomas splint
   Lower leg and foot — inflatable leg splint (if not available tie legs together and splint as best you can)
4 Transportation:
   For back and pelvis injuries — use a lifting frame
   Neck fractures — support head with the neck in extension
   If a lifting frame is not available at least three persons are necessary to transfer the patient in one straight piece

ASSESSMENT

1 *History taking* from the patient (and bystanders and ambulance men). This should include:
   Details of injury
   Present symptoms
   Past history of injury
   Having taken the history YOU MUST WRITE IT DOWN
2 *Undress patients* — if necessary cut clothes off.
3 *Examine* — the physical signs of a fracture are:
   Swelling and bruising and loss of function
   Deformity and shortening
   Local bone tenderness (abnormal movement and crepitus may be found but should not be sought after)
4 *Exclude anatomical complications of fractures*
Vascular complications:
   note skin colour and movements
   test for sensation and movements

29

Neurological complications:
    test for sensation and movements
Visceral lesions may complicate fractures of pelvis, spine or
    chest.
5 *Examine for associated fracture patterns*
Fractures of the calcaneus are associated with crush fractures of
    the spine.
Dislocation of the hip in a road traffic accident is associated
    with a knee injury (Fig. 2.1).

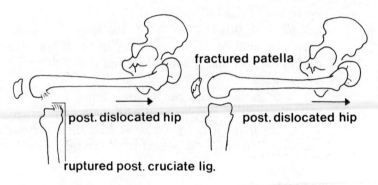

fractured patella

post. dislocated hip   post. dislocated hip

ruptured post. cruciate lig.

Fig. 2.1. Dashboard injuries

Head injuries are associated with cervical spine lesions.
Having examined the patient YOU MUST WRITE DOWN YOUR
    FINDINGS.
6 *X-rays are mandatory*
An X-ray is essential to exclude a suspected fracture.
A fracture cannot be defined clinically with sufficient accuracy
    to permit adequate treatment.
An A-P and lateral X-ray are necessary. These must be centred
    on the area of suspected fracture. The X-ray should include
    the joint above and below the fracture.
If one is not sure of the anatomy of the epiphyses in a child the
    other limb can be X-rayed.
If a fracture is not shown on the routine A-P and lateral views
    it is reasonable to ask for further oblique films.
Some crack or undisplaced fractures are not easily demons-

trated initially. It is wise to ask for repeat films some ten days later when the fracture is easier to see.

Patients with multiple injuries should always have an X-ray of chest and pelvis.

Patients with head injuries should always have X-rays of the cervical spine. Cervical spine X-rays must always show the seventh cervical vertebra.

OUTLINE OF MANAGEMENT OF MULTIPLE INJURIES

First aid at accident site:
  Clear airway — of debris and tongue
                — extend neck and support chin
  Treat hypovolaemic shock — by transfusion if necessary
  Stop external bleeding by pressure bandaging
  Splint fractures
  Arrange transport — if possible use a lifting frame
In hospital — transfer direct to triage (or intensive care) area.
Check first aid measures. Then organise emergency treatment and assessment.

Respiratory problems
Clear airway — if necessary intubate
Close open sucking wounds
Treat pneumothorax — intercostal drain to underwater seal
Treat haemothorax — by aspiration and drainage
Manage flail segments and paradoxical respiration — by intubation and positive pressure respiration.

Cardiovascular problems
Treat and minimise the effects of hypovolaemic shock;
  Organise intravenous infusion:
    initially Ringer's lactate or plasma preparation
    preferably blood of patient's group
  Monitor infusion:
    by central venous pressure monitor
    by checking urine output
    by estimating clinically from the number of fractures and the size of the wounds

Chapter 2

Head injury
Note state of consciousness
CNS signs particularly:
   pupils
   localising signs
A continual check is made of these signs and they are charted.
A deterioration of neurological state may be an indication for
operative treatment.

Abdominal lesions
They represent as persistent bleeding and later may cause
peritonitis.
Note: bruising and clothing imprints on abdomen;
   increasing distension especially in children;
   bowel sounds and localised tenderness are not found in a
      severely shocked patient;
   peritoneal aspiration or lavage is a useful investigation.
If an intra-abdominal injury is suspected a laparotomy is undertaken as soon as possible.

Fractures
Fractures always require splintage no matter how sick the
patient. Simple and quick emergency treatment involves the
use of padded plaster slabs and skeletal traction devices. All
fractures can be adequately controlled by such methods in the
short-term. Compound fractures require adequate operative
debridement as soon as possible, as do other lacerations and
wounds (see p. 44).

Examination
During resuscitation and when the patient is stable all clothing
should be removed. The patient is thoroughly examined clinically and notes made of the examination. The examination can
be anatomical — head, chest, abdomen, limbs and back; and
then systematic — cardiovascular and neurological.

X-rays
X-rays of chest and pelvis must be taken in all cases of multiple
injury. If a skull X-ray is indicated then an X-ray of the
cervical spine is also indicated.

TREATMENT OF FRACTURES

First aid (p. 29)
Treatment of other injuries and of hypovolaemic shock (p. 31)
Reduction if necessary:
  by manipulation
  by traction
  by operation
Fixation, if necessary:
  by slings and bandages
  by plaster
  by traction
  by internal fixation
Mobilisation and restoration of function of joints and soft tissues
Rehabilitation

It is not possible or necessary to reduce or fix some fractures. Stable, crush fractures of the spine or fractures of the pelvis are such fractures. These patients are treated symptomatically with rest until their acute symptoms subside. They are then prescribed mobilising exercises until fit to resume their normal occupations.

Manipulative reduction
This method will afford a satisfactory (but not always anatomical reduction) of most fractures. If possible, fracture manipulation should:
  be accomplished under general anaesthesia;
  be followed immediately by check X-ray.
They are best performed in hospital. The only manoeuvres that will be described are those for Colles' fracture (p. 70) and shoulder dislocation (p. 95).

Slings and bandages (Fig. 2.2)
Slings are used for immobilisation of upper limb fractures. They can be used in conjunction with a body bandage or even the patient's own clothing. A broad arm sling with a well-fitting T-shirt over the top is adequate immobilisation for an undisplaced fracture of the neck of the humerus in a child. Common types of sling in use are:

33

broad arm sling

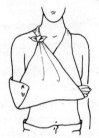

collar and cuff

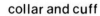
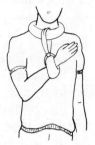

St John's sling

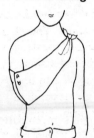

sling under clothes

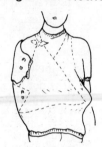

Fig. 2.2.   Different types of sling

broad arm sling (triangular) for shoulder injuries;
collar and cuff sling for elbow injuries;
high or St John sling for hand injuries and elevating the
    forearm.
A figure-of-eight bandage is useful for a fractured clavicle in
conjunction with a broad arm sling.

Tractions
When traction is applied to a fractured limb it acts in two
ways: directly on the fracture site pulling the broken ends apart
and thus into alignment. Secondly it acts on the muscles about
the fracture, overcoming muscle spasm. In due course the
muscles form a tube which confines the fracture permitting
union in reasonable alignment.
    The types of traction to be considered:
        skin traction
        skeletal traction

traction using a Thomas splint
modified Hamilton Russell traction
skull traction

Skin traction involves the use of strapping extensions applied to the lower limbs. The extensions are of elastoplast and their adhesiveness is assisted by using tinct-benz co.

A simple form of traction can be used to rest a painful limb following injury. The patient lies flat in bed with the end of the bed raised. A weight is applied to the affected limb by the use of skin traction. Such traction can also be used for patients with back pain and acute sciatica.

Fractures of the femur in small children (under three years of age) can be treated by gallows traction. The child lies flat on its back and the legs are suspended vertically by skin extensions. A weight is attached to the extensions by a pulley as shown in the diagram (Fig. 2.3). It is wise to use pulleys and leave the buttocks on the bed; it is thus possible to know how much traction is applied to the lower limb. Unfortunately it is possible to cause ischaemic problems of the lower leg or traction nerve injuries if too much weight is applied.

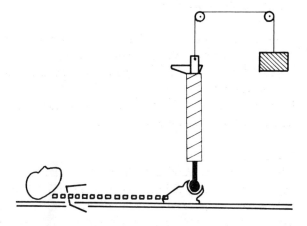

Fig. 2.3. Gallows traction

Older children with fractured femurs can be immobilised in skin traction and a Thomas splint.

Skeletal traction involves the use of a pin placed through a bone. When treating fractures of the shaft of the femur in adults, the upper end of the tibia is usually used; the pin is inserted in close relation to the tibial tubercle. This has the advantage of permitting greater weight to be applied to the limb and also it is more permanent as skin extensions tend to peel off after a few weeks. It must be remembered that in growing children the pin should never be placed near the tibial tubercle as this is an actively growing epiphyseal plate. The pin may also be placed through the lower end of the femur.

Fractures of the tibia can be treated with traction via pins placed either through the lower end of the tibia or through the calcaneus.

The Thomas splint can be used for treating fractures of the femur. It consists of a leather ring at its upper end which is designed to fit snugly around the groin and impinge on the ischial tuberosity. Attached to this are metal extensions joined at the lower end which fit on either side of the lower leg and below the foot. Traction can be applied via skin extensions or via a skeletal pin.

Fixed traction requires the use of a Thomas splint. The traction cords are tied to the end of the splint after exerting

force transmitted to buttock

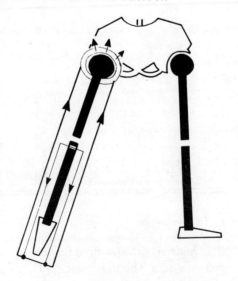

Fig. 2.4. Fixed traction

traction on the limb. A closed system is thus formed; traction from the cords is transmitted back up to the groin and the ischial tuberosity via the bars of the splint (Fig. 2.4).

This has the advantage of allowing the patient to be nursed comfortably and simply and be transported easily. Furthermore, the system is isometric, there is little danger of distracting the fracture. However, the cords must be kept taut and the ring of the splint must fit snugly into the groin. The system must therefore be used with great care in acute injuries when the patient has a swollen thigh.

Sliding (balanced) traction. In this form of traction the traction weight is balanced by the weight of the patient sliding down a slope. The slope is usually provided by elevating the end of the bed. In fact all traction, but fixed traction in a splint, can be described and classified as sliding or balanced traction.

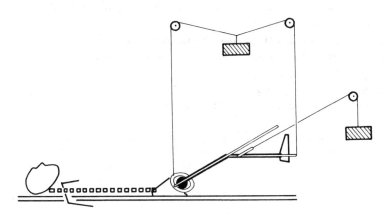

Fig. 2.5. Sliding traction with Thomas splint

In the system in Fig. 2.5 the Thomas splint is merely a vehicle to elevate the leg and permit easy nursing. A knee piece is attached which maintains the knee in flexion. This helps prevent external rotation flop and also relaxes the peroneal nerve. The knee is more comfortable and knee stiffness less of a problem after union of the fracture.

Modified Hamilton Russell traction is a most useful form of traction. This can be applied by a skeletal pin through the tibial tubercle. A support is applied to the lower leg. A sling is applied under the thigh to support it. Traction is applied via the tibial tubercle and also via the end of the leg support by a system of pulleys much as shown in the diagram. This is a very useful form of traction for treating people with lesions around the hip joint and upper end of the femur. Rotation can be adequately controlled and the apparatus is comfortable (Fig. 2.6).

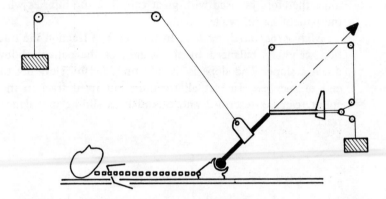

Fig. 2.6. Adapted Hamilton Russell traction

Skull traction is used for fractures and dislocation of the cervical spine. It is best applied via Barton's tongs. These are inserted into the outer table of the skull in the region of the parietal eminence (in line with the external auditory meatus) (Fig. 2.7).

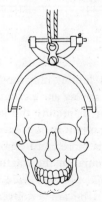

Fig. 2.7. Skull calipers

The patient can be nursed in a turning bed and traction maintained — holding the cervical spine in alignment. Skull traction can be continued satisfactorily for months if necessary (Fig. 2.8).

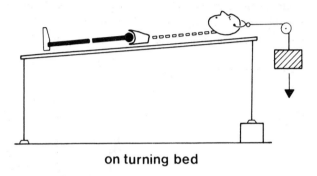

on turning bed

Fig. 2.8. Skull traction

PLASTER OF PARIS IMMOBILISATION

Plaster is the most useful material for splinting fractures. Other materials are used but each has its limitations and complications. Plaster of Paris is calcium sulphate. The anhydrous powder is impregnated into bandages. When wet the anhydrous form of calcium sulphate is transformed into the hydrated form. This sets firmly with the evolution of heat.

Principles of using plaster
Clinically it is necessary to immobilise the joint above and below the fracture. This is the only way to control rotation in unstable fractures.

The plaster should be 'moulded' to obtain three-point fixation of a fracture — preferably in two planes (Fig. 2.9). Use is made of the intact soft tissues on the concave side of the fracture.

When reducing a fracture the position in which it is stable is determined. The plaster is applied and moulded to hold the fracture in that stable reduced position. If there is not a stable position then another method of fixation may be necessary.

Plaster is best applied as slabs when fixing acute fractures and dislocations. If signs of compression occur the plaster is

39

more easily split. If the patient is allowed home after emergency treatment, only slabs should be used.

A complete plaster should only be used for acute cases in special circumstances. If it is so used, it must be split, and the split must pass through the padding and dressings as well as the plaster.

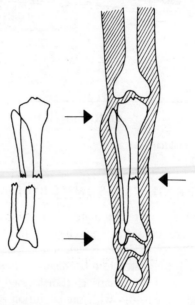

Fig. 2.9. Moulded long-leg plaster

The application of plaster
The limb must be held in the correct position. Only the flats of the hands are used, to prevent local pressure on the plaster.

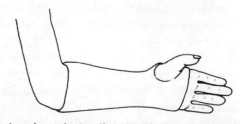

extends only to distal palmar crease

Fig. 2.10. Below-elbow plaster

A single layer of plaster wool is applied smoothly and continuously — double layers can be used over bony prominences. A thin layer of foam rubber may be used at these pressure sites (Fig. 2.11).

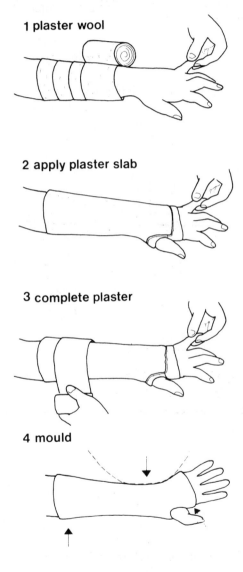

1 plaster wool

2 apply plaster slab

3 complete plaster

4 mould

Fig. 2.11. Application of below-elbow plaster

Plaster bandage rolls are immersed in luke warm water until all bubbles have ceased. The roll is gently squeezed out securing the free end. The plaster is applied as a single continuous layer smoothing out as applied. Plaster slabs are used strategically to reinforce. The complete plaster is kept still and elevated preventing local pressure indentations as it dries.

The patient is given specific instructions:

Keep limb elevated for twenty-four hours — the arm in a sling, the leg on pillows or on a couch or bed;

Keep plaster dry;

Move all movable joints above and below the plaster;

Attend immediately if swelling or discoloration of skin or if symptoms of tingling or numbness occur;

Attend next day for plaster check.

Common types of plaster

Below-elbow plaster extends from below the elbow to the level of the metacarpo-phalangeal joints; these are marked by the distal skin crease on the palm (see Figs. 2.10 and 2.11).

The plaster must not extend beyond this skin crease otherwise the metacarpo-phalangeal joints will be fixed in extension and become stiff.

A scaphoid plaster is used for scaphoid fractures and lesions about the base of the thumb. It extends from below the elbow to the distal palmar crease with the wrist in some dorsi-flexion. The plaster extends over the thumb to the inter-phalangeal joint.

An above-elbow plaster is used for forearm fractures. It extends from just distal to the axilla to the distal palmar

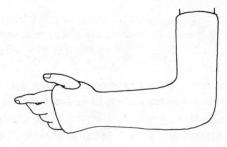

Fig. 2.12. Above-elbow POP

crease. The elbow is immobilised in ninety degrees of flexion. The wrist position depends on the fracture — extremes of dorsi-flexion and palmar flexion are avoided (Fig. 2.12).

An above-knee plaster is used to immobilise fractures of the tibia and fibula. It extends from the groin to the metatarsal heads. The knee is immobilised in about twenty degrees of flexion and the ankle fixed at right angles (Fig. 2.13a).

It is important not to immobilise the ankle in any degree of plantar flexion (equinus). An ankle stiff in equinus is very difficult to correct.

A plaster cylinder extends from the groin to the malleoli. It is used for knee injuries. It requires careful padding at the lower end (Fig. 2.13b).

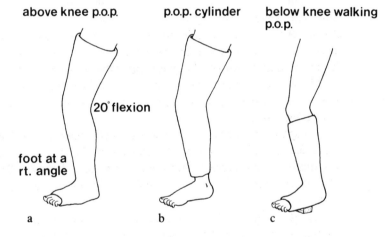

above knee p.o.p.   **p.o.p. cylinder**   **below knee walking p.o.p.**

20° flexion

foot at a
rt. angle

a   b   c

Fig. 2.13a–c.   Different kinds of leg plaster

A below-knee plaster extends from just below the knee to the metatarsal heads. It is used for ankle and foot injuries. The ankle must be at right angles and the foot in neutral position (Fig. 2.13c).

If the plaster is required for metatarsal and toe fractures, a platform can be constructed to fit under the toes for support.

Weight bearing can be allowed after a protective heel or boot is applied to the foot portion. Weight bearing should be encouraged as soon as possible to improve the circulation in the limb and at the fracture site and to decrease oedema.

A *cast brace* is a particular type of weight-bearing plaster for the lower limb which has been adapted to permit movement at the knee and at the ankle. It is used when healing of the fracture has reached such a stage that there is some inherent stability. A total contact plaster is applied to the lower limb and a hinge is inserted at the knee and at the ankle. Its effectiveness depends on the fact that at body temperatures the soft tissues act as fluid and are not compressible. The total contact plaster applied to the fracture will subject it to hydrostatic pressure and maintain its position satisfactorily. Adjustable plastic splints have now been developed and have a similar function. In many centres these have largely replaced the original plaster cast braces.

The main disadvantages of treating fractures in plaster are:

Prolonged immobilisation causes stiffness in joints and oedema and other circulatory problems in the limbs.

Plasters are heavy and inconvenient. Old people in particular find them difficult to manage.

They tend to disintegrate and fragment, especially if wet.

Some fractures are not adequately controlled in plaster.

However, there are advantages:

Plasters are safe if properly applied.

The immobilisation is simple and adequate for most fractures.

Application of plaster does not require expensive or sophisticated facilities.

OPERATIONS ON FRACTURES

The indications for operating on fractures are:

Compound fractures

Treatment of the complications of fractures

Failure of fixation by plaster or traction

Necessity for an anatomical reduction

Desirability of early mobilisation

Pathological fractures in long bones

Compound fractures

A compound fracture is an absolute indication for operation. It is necessary to treat the wound to prevent infection. Having

done that the fracture is immobilised and allowed to unite. Compound fractures are liable to be infected by:
Pyogenic staphylococci from the patient or his attendants;
Mixed contaminating organisms introduced from without;
Anaerobic organisms — tetanus and gas gangrene.
There are three types of compound fracture:
Type I: from within — a bone spike penetrates the skin. There is often little soft tissue damage and less risk of infection.
Type II: fractures associated with extensive skin damage but little deep tissue damage.
Type III: fractures with serious wounds from without and a considerable amount of dead tissue. There may be foreign material deeply implanted. These fractures require careful and extensive debridement.

The management of compound fractures
First aid measures, treatment of hypovolaemic shock and other injuries.
Prevent infection:
tetanus prophylaxis
antibiotics
(debridement)
Operation in a theatre under general anaesthesia:
wash and irrigate wound and shave skin;
debridement:
skin — wound edges are excised and obviously dead skin removed;
fat amd fascia — all damaged and contaminated tissue removed;
muscle — all damaged and contaminated tissue removed until bright red, bleeding and contracting muscle remains;
bone fragments — small loose fragments are removed, large and attached fragments remain;
nerves and arteries — may be repaired.
The fracture is reduced and held by:
traction
plaster
external fixation device (internal fixation is rarely used in

compound fractures because of the danger of potentiating infection)

Skin closure:

primary closure only in Types I and II compound fractures within eight hours of injury;

delayed closure in Type III and other fractures over eight hours old. Skin grafting is usually necessary a week or two after the initial operation. After eight hours a compound fracture is very likely to be an infected fracture.

Post-operative:

fracture is immobilised and elevated;

antibiotics are given intravenously.

De-gloving injuries

A crushing or rolling type of injury can cause the skin and subcutaneous fascia to be stripped off the deep fascia and so lose its blood supply. Cases have been described where the skin has been peeled off the hand and foot like a glove.

There can be extensive loss of skin from these injuries. They can be treated by defatting the affected skin and replacing it as a graft. Frequently it dies and skin grafting is necessary.

Many severe compound fractures are associated with areas of skin damaged in this way. Care must be taken to recognise this possibility and manage it.

INTERNAL FIXATION

Internal fixation of fractures by operation permits an accurate anatomical reduction of the fracture. This is particularly important for fractures about joints. Secondly it assures firm accurate fixation of the fracture. This in turn permits early mobilisation of joints and soft tissues and reduces the time of convalescence. Compression together of the two fracture ends is the best way to obtain firm fixation.

The materials used for internal fixation are usually metallic alloys. They must have the following properties:

1 The alloy must be strong enough;

2 It must have a high fatigue limit;

3 It must not be corroded by body fluids;

4 The components must not set up an electric couple between themselves. If both components are made of metal, the alloy used must be identical;
5 It must not set up an immune reaction in the body tissue.

It is found that the strength, resistance to fatigue, and resistance to corrosion also depend on the surface of the implant and on its design. Other important factors include:
1 The presence of an inert oxide film over the surface of an implant. The film will prevent corrosion.
2 The surface should be smooth. The implant should have rounded edges and screw holes. Care must be taken to prevent scratching and damaging the implant during its insertion. Notches, scratches and sharp prominences act as stress risers causing concentration of stresses. This weakens the material and reduces its resistance to fatigue failure.
3 Impurities in the metal must be avoided as corrosion will start there.
4 The components of the implant must be fitted tightly and fixed firmly to the bone to prevent fretting corrosion.
5 Infection must be avoided.

Three metal alloys are in common use for the construction of implants:

Stainless steel — SMO 18/8
  Iron 70%
  Chromium 17%
  Nickel 10%
  Molybdenum 2.4%
Vitallium
  Chromium 65%
  Cobalt 30%
  Molybdenum 5%
Titanium alloy
  Aluminium 6%
  Vanadium 4%

IMPLANTS

Design consideration of implants:
1 They must be strong enough and compact enough to fit within the fracture anatomy.

2 They must not interfere with normal fracture repair processes.

3 The operation to insert the implant must be performed easily by the average surgeon in a reasonable time. If a procedure takes over two hours infection is likely.

4 The device must permit anatomical reduction and hold the fracture under some degree of compression.

Bone screws
These compress the fragments together. Lagging of screws is an advantage as the screw threads do not separate the fragments.

Wires
These should be used on the tensile surface and compress the fragments together. Encirclage wires will tend to interrupt the blood supply of the bone fragments.

Plates
These should be used on the tensile surfaces of bones and will hold fractures under compression. Compression plating will appose the fracture ends even more closely and hold the fracture rigidly.

Intramedullary devices
Impact in the medullary canal.

The Kuntscher nail used for fractured femurs has a clover leaf cross-section. It is relatively strong and resists bending. There is little resistance however, to torsion and this depends on the interdigitation of the fracture fragments (Fig. 2.14).

Flexible rods act by affording internal three point fixation.

Devices for fractures of the neck of the femur
Subcapital fractures
    can be fixed by two or three threaded nails (Fig 2.15a);
    can be fixed by a nail and plate to control rotation and
        permit collapse of the neck (Fig. 2.15b).
Displaced subcapital fractures have such a high incidence of avascular necrosis that the head of the femur is often replaced by a prosthesis (Fig. 2.15c).

Pertrochanteric fractures are best fixed by a nail and plate.

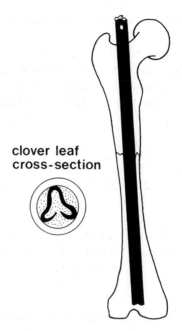

clover leaf
cross-section

Fig. 2.14. Kuntscher nail

If they are comminuted they tend to collapse and a sliding nail can be used (Fig. 2.15b).

PHYSIOTHERAPY AND OCCUPATIONAL THERAPY

Both these help restore function to the injured patient.

The physiotherapist works using exercise therapy and various physical methods to restore movement and muscle function and reduce oedema.

The occupational therapist concentrates more on the restoration of function for activities used in ordinary life and in work. She is also an expert on mechanical aids. During the healing process a therapist can:

encourage movements of all free joints;

assist mobility by teaching crutch walking and weight bearing in plaster;

encourage static excercises of limbs in plaster and band-

Chapter 2

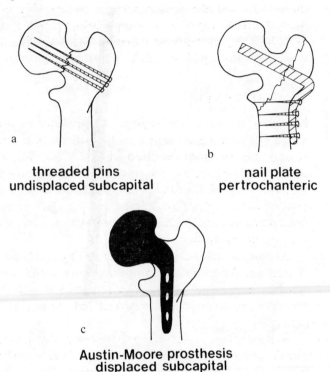

a

**threaded pins
undisplaced subcapital**

b

**nail plate
pertrochanteric**

c

**Austin-Moore prosthesis
displaced subcapital**

Fig. 2.15a–c. Fixation of fractures of the femur neck

ages. This will tend to reduce muscle wasting and improve circulation;

encourage an apprehensive and depressed patient by her
attention.

A fractured limb after healing may show stiffness due to fibrosis
of damaged muscles, joint adhesions and prolonged immobilisation.

Immobilisation and reflex inhibition of muscles due to
trauma may cause muscle wasting. Impaired circulation may be
a cause of oedema. Correction of these takes time and patience
and encouragement to perform active exercises and gradually
restore normal function.

Patients after injury become unfit for physical work. General exercises in a gymnasium are necessary to restore such
fitness. Patients after fracture lose ability to work and perform
normal activities. Many have to be encouraged to undertake

these tasks and the process takes a considerable time. An occupational therapist is trained to help patients and advise them how to perform these activities. She is also in a position to advise when a patient is fit to return to his normal work.

REHABILITATION

It is unfortunate that rehabilitation is a word that means different things to different people. Some patients are restored to normal after fractures and some are not. Those who are (and accept the fact) have no problems. Those who are 'not normal' are left with some disability. The latter can be divided into two groups: those with a mild disability, i.e. who can return to their previous occupations, and those with a severe disability who are unable to work as before.

Almost all disabled patients (except with significant mental or intellectual impairment) can peform some useful work. Disabled patients should be encouraged to perform useful work so that they can retain their self respect and the respect of their colleagues.

Rehabilitation means advising a patient that a permanent disability is not correctable. It also means finding him work he is capable of doing and compensating him adequately for loss of wages and for the loss of ability to perform normal tasks and his usual recreations.

Rehabilitation is the responsibility not only of doctors but also society as a whole. Societies often do not appreciate their responsibility.

A doctor is requested to give reports on patients as to fitness for work and also to assess residual disability. This is usually a difficult task and often impossible. The only consolation is that any doctor knows more about it than any layman.

Residual disability is assessed in terms of pathological anatomy (such as proportionate loss of a lower limb). Various tables have been constructed giving percentage disability for particular anatomical lesions.

Fitness for work is difficult to assess. Fortunately most patients will admit when they are fit to return to work. An occasional patient will not admit when he is to fit to return to work and this can cause problems. Such patients are best examined by an anonymous panel.

3 Hand Injuries

FINGER INJURIES

** Soft tissue lacerations
*** Digital nerve injuries
*** The non-viable finger
*** Tendon injuries

Finger injuries are very common. They can cause prolonged disability and are worth careful treatment. Aims of treatment are that the fingers:

must be mobile;

must have adequate sensibility.

If they are rigid or anaesthetic after treatment they are a nuisance and better amputated. With the thumb, however, all length must be maintained even if it has to be converted to a rigid post. Sensibility must also be restored.

These aims are accomplished by meticulous management of the soft tissue component of the injury, by careful and precise debridement, and appropriate closure of the skin.

Fingers must only be immobilised for a short time. The position of the immobilisation is critical (Fig. 3.1):

metacarpo-phalangeal joints at 90°;

interphalangeal joints in extension or only slight flexion.

Finger joints should be mobilised by gentle active movements as soon as possible. It is better to have a mobile, crooked finger

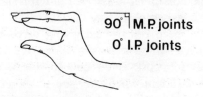

90° M.P. joints
0° I.P. joints

Fig. 3.1. Position of immobilization of the hand

52

than a stiff straight one. It is justifiable to operate and fix finger fractures so that the early movement is possible.

** **Soft tissue lacerations**
These can be:
    clean incisions
    crushing injuries associated with bursting of the skin. The damage to soft tissues is difficult to determine
Examination should exclude injuries:
of tendons
of digital nerves
X-ray will exclude associated fractures and dislocations.

Management
Prevent infection:
    tetanus prophylaxis
    use aseptic precautions
    clean and debride wound to remove contaminants
    use antibiotics if the wound is at all extensive or contaminated
Closure:
    primary suture only if clean and incised
    dress and allow to heal secondarily if contaminated or a crushing injury
    skin graft if extensive skin loss (a partial amputation may be more appropriate)

*** **Digital nerve injuries**
These are best treated by primary suture unless there is severe injury or a badly contaminated wound. Magnification, general anaesthesia and a tourniquet are essential.

*** **The non-viable finger**
This should be amputated. The sites of amputation of a finger are:
    peripheral to the distal interphalangeal joint to permit skin closure;
    through the DIP joint or just proximal to it (distal to the sublimis insertions so that the PIP joint can flex);

through the base of the proximal phalanx to preserve breadth of the hand.

All the length of the thumb must be preserved. The most unlikely thumb remnants can be used for reconstruction.

It is possible to repair digital veins and arteries by micro-vascular surgery and thus make a non-viable finger viable. Nerves, tendons, bone and skin also require repair and must function well to make such a procedure worthwhile. If the patient is left with a stiff or anaesthetic finger after microvascular surgery, he would still be better off with an amputation.

Tendon injuries
** 1 Extensor tendon injuries
*** 2 Flexor tendon injuries
* 3 Mallet finger
** 4 Boutonnière deformity

On laceration of a tendon the two ends retract. In order for healing to occur the severed endings must be apposed. After apposition of the severed ends, the area of the laceration is surrounded by a blood clot which will organise. The organising tissue contains fibroblasts which are derived from the peritenon. These fibroblasts form new collagen which fuses with that in the remaining ends of the tendon. A mass of 'tendon callus' results. In due course the tendon will remodel. This remodelling occurs when activity is resumed. The majority of tendon lacerations will heal provided the two ends are adequately apposed.

** *Extensor tendon injuries of the hand*
These should be treated as follows:
1 The wound is explored under a torniquet with the patient anaesthetised in an operating theatre.
2 The tendon ends are sutured. This repair should be as meticulous as possible using non absorbable sutures.
3 Following this the finger will require to be splinted for about two or three weeks with the site of repair relaxed.
4 Following this, graduated exercises are required as remod-elling of the tendon and resolution of stiffness of the finger occurs.

*** *Flexor tendon injuries*

The management of injuries to the flexor tendons of the hand is more complicated.

The flexor sublimis tendon lies superficial to the profundus in the palm. As they pass to the finger they are enclosed in an osseofibrous tunnel formed by the fibrous flexor sheath and the proximal phalanx. The tendons are in close apposition in this tunnel. In the region of the proximal interphalangeal joint the sublimis tendon splits and is inserted into the middle phalanx by extensions which embrace the profundus tendon. The profundus tendon continues to be inserted into the distal phalanx.

If the tendons are cut in the osseofibrous tunnel and repaired without special care a mass of granulation tissue will form. Normal function will not resume after resolution of this mass. The treatment depends on the anatomical site of the tendon injury. Three zones are described (Fig. 3.2):

1 The flexor profundus may be injured on its own distal to the osseofibrous tunnel (the distal zone).

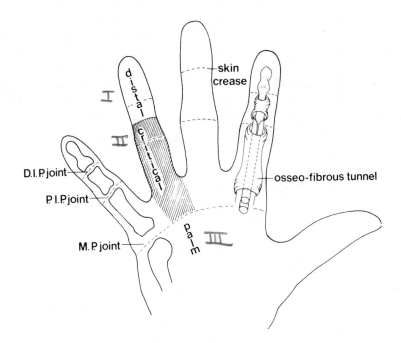

Fig. 3.2. Flexor sheaths of fingers. Tendon insertion

2 Both tendons may be injured in the osseofibrous tunnel (the critical zone or 'no man's land').

3 Tendon injury in the palm.

The actual technique of suturing the tendons is critical. These injuries are much best managed by a patient, fastidious surgeon using fine instruments and very fine suturing material and an operating microscope. They should not be treated by the casual operator.

Using such modern techniques the results obtained by primary suture of the flexor tendons are such as would have been considered impossible in the past. However, if special facilities are not available or the wound is dirty or of long standing, it is wise to clean and debride the wound as is routinely done and allow skin healing to take place. After the skin is healed the patient can be transferred and tendon repair performed at leisure. This would consist of either direct suture of the tendons or more probably excision of them and a tendon graft. The results of this sort of operation are less certain than those of early primary suture.

* *Mallet finger*

A mallet finger results from disruption of the extensor tendon attachment to the distal phalanx (Fig. 3.3). The patient is aware of knocking her finger, as whilst making beds. The finger takes up an attitude of flexion at the distal interphalangeal joint. Usually the lesion is through the fibrous attachment of tendon to bone — occasionally a bone fragment is avulsed.

Treatment is by splinting the joint in extension — a variety of splints have been designed for this purpose. Very occasionally a large bone fragment is avulsed and inverted, only these patients benefit from operation and fixation.

Children can develop this deformity after injury. The lesion is a separation of the epiphysis and growth plate from the distal phalanx. The treatment is splintage (Fig. 3.3).

** *Boutonnière deformity*

A Boutonnière deformity follows disruption of the central slip of the extensor expansion which is inserted into the middle phalanx. A flexion deformity occurs at the proximal interphalangeal joint with hyperextension at the distal joint. It is an

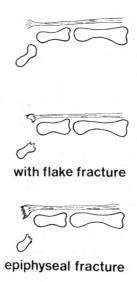

with flake fracture

epiphyseal fracture

Fig. 3.3. Mallet finger

ugly disabling deformity (Fig. 3.4). Unfortunately it is difficult
to diagnose early. If the lesion is closed and seen early —
splinting of the proximal interphalangeal joint in extension is
the best treatment. (If the lesion is open or seen late operation
is indicated.)

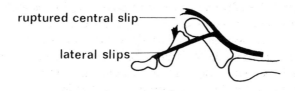

ruptured central slip

lateral slips

Fig. 3.4. Boutonnière deformity

FRACTURES OF FINGERS

** Fractures of distal phalanx
*** Shaft fractures of middle and proximal phalanges
*** Avulsion fractures
*** Fracture dislocations
** Childrens' finger fractures

Chapter 3

** Fractures of distal phalanx

These usually result from crushing injuries. Their management depends on the degree of soft tissue damage, which requires meticulous treatment. The fractures are adequately immobilised by a bulky dressing. When the soft tissues have healed so has the fracture.

*** Fractures of the shafts of the middle and proximal phalanges

* *Undisplaced*

These are usually stable and only simple splintage is required. This can be achieved by intermittent strapping to an adjacent uninjured finger. Early movement is encouraged (Fig. 3.5). It is important to ensure that the fracture is undisplaced. It is sometimes difficult to determine on X-ray whether there is a rotational displacement. However, this can be determined by looking at the tips of the fingers and making sure that they are in reasonable alignment (Fig. 3.6). Furthermore if the fingers are flexed they will be seen to appose the base of the thenar eminence each individually. A finger with a rotational deformity will not do this.

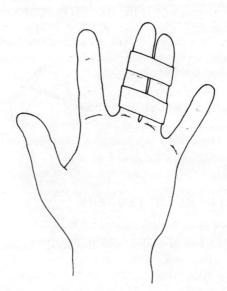

Fig. 3.5. Intermittent strapping of fingers

58

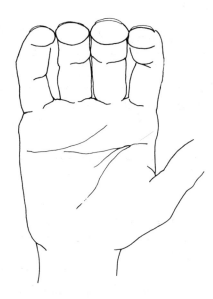

Fig. 3.6. Normal relationship, fingertips

*** *Displaced*
These fractures are difficult to manage and they are often compound. They may be reduced and immobilised on a plaster slab with the finger flexed to $90°$ at the metacarpo-phalangeal joint and extended at the interphalangeal joints (Fig. 3.7). However, in order to obtain an accurate reduction and permit early movements operation and internal fixation of these fractures is often a worthwhile procedure.

*** **Avulsion fractures**
In association with mallet finger (see above).
In association with separation of the volar plate from the base of the middle phalanx (Fig. 3.8).
In association with separation of the collateral ligaments.
   If the fragments are small they can be ignored and the finger treated by intermittent strapping and early movement. If the fragment is large it should be replaced at operation and the joint mobilised as soon as possible.

*** **Fracture dislocation (or subluxations) of the finger**
These tend to be unstable and frequently present late. They are

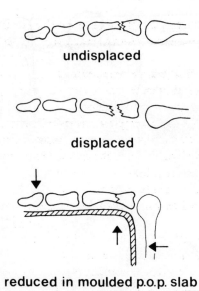

Fig. 3.7. Fractures of the proximal phalanx

very difficult to manage (Fig. 3.8). Open reduction and internal fixation is the ideal treatment, but unfortunately is not often possible. Patients presenting late are probably best treated with intermittent strapping and early mobilisation. It is better to have a mobile crooked finger than a stiff straight one.

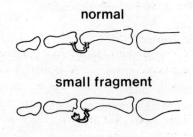

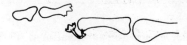

Fig. 3.8. Avulsion fractures of the volar plate

Childrens' finger fractures

** *Greenstick fractures* occur in the shaft of phalanges. These can be simply reduced and held with splints.

** *A fracture near the growth plate of the base of the proximal phalanx of the little finger* occurs commonly. The finger is displaced away from the hand in an ulnar direction. The fracture requires reduction. This reduction can be maintained with intermittent strapping.

Dislocations of fingers

** *Interphalangeal joint dislocations*
These can be simply reduced and the finger immobilised with intermittent strapping. If there is an associated fracture the prognosis may be poor.

*** *Metacarpo-phalangeal joint dislocation*
This injury usually reduces spontaneously. If it presents clinically it is often complicated. The volar plate may be interposed between the articular surfaces. This may prevent reduction or make it imperfect. Operation is required to reduce the dislocation.

*** **Gamekeeper's thumb** (Fig. 3.9)
This injury results from damage to the ulnar collateral ligament of the metacarpo-phalangeal joint of the thumb. It is quite a

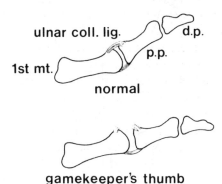

Fig. 3.9. Lesion of the ulnar collateral ligament

Chapter 3

common sporting injury, particularly in basketball and rugby football. There may be an associated flake fracture from the head of the metacarpal or the base of proximal phalanx. If the lesion is missed, the thumb becomes unstable and tends to give way on pressure. It then requires an operation to reconstruct the collateral ligament. It is best to diagnose this lesion as soon as possible and immobilise the thumb in a scaphoid plaster. Often the two portions of the ligament become separated by the adductor pollicis tendon, in which case, open operation is the best treatment.

FRACTURES OF METACARPALS

   * Fractures of neck of fifth metacarpal
  ** Fractures of shafts of metacarpals
  ** Fractures of base of first metacarpal
 *** Carpo-metacarpal dislocations

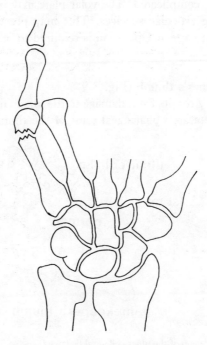

Fig. 3.10.   Fracture of the neck of the fifth metacarpal

* **Fracture of the neck of the fifth metacarpal (Boxer's fracture)**
(Fig. 3.10)
These are common fractures which occur after striking with a
closed fist. The head of the metacarpal is forced into flexion. A
considerable amount of flexion is acceptable and reduction is
rarely necessary. Patients can be treated symptomatically with
a crêpe bandage. Usually a volar slab plaster with the wrist in
dorsi-flexion is required. The fingers are left free except for
intermittent strapping between the ring and little finger.

** **Fractures of the shafts of the metacarpals**
Undisplaced oblique fractures are common. They can be treated
symptomatically with either a crêpe bandage or a cock-up
plaster.

Occasionally a spiral fracture can be associated with rupture
of the transverse metacarpal ligament. The fracture is unstable
and the finger rotated. This should be checked for by flexing
the finger and noting its relationship to the base of the thenar
eminence.

Severe injuries can cause multiple unstable fractures of the
metacarpals. They can be associated with carpo-metacarpal dislocations. They are often compound and complicated injuries.
These fractures are best treated by operation and internal
fixation.

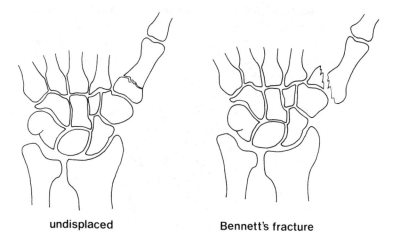

undisplaced   Bennett's fracture

Fig. 3.11. Fracture of the base of the first metacarpal

Chapter 3

** **Fractures of the base of the first metacarpal** (Fig. 3.11)
A fracture near the base of the first metacarpal is common. A considerable degree of angulation can be accepted. This fracture is treated by immobilisation in a scaphoid plaster.

*** *Bennett's fracture* is a fracture through the articular surface of the first metacarpal with lateral displacement of the metacarpal shaft (Fig. 3.11). It is very difficult to obtain an accurate reduction of this fracture by closed means. It is probably best fixed by percutaneous pinning using an image intensifier.

*** **Carpo-metacarpal dislocations**
These occur after severe injuries — often compound and associated with other fractures. They are best treated by open reduction and internal fixation.

INJURIES OF THE CARPUS

*** Fractures of the scaphoid
*** Carpal subluxations
* Flake fractures of the carpus
*** Fracture of the hook of the hamate

Fractures of the scaphoid
The scaphoid transmits force from the radial side of the hand to the radius. Furthermore it is a link bone acting as a connecting rod between the proximal and distal rows of the carpus. It is associated with flexion and extension movements of the wrist and rotates with movements of the thumb.

It has a critical blood supply. The distal pole is vascular. The main nutrient artery however enters about the waist and fractures proximal to it may be complicated by non-union or avascular necrosis of its proximal fragment. Displaced fractures are even more likely to suffer these complications.

Undisplaced fractures of the scaphoid are difficult to see on X-ray. Oblique views should be taken as a routine. A patient who shows wrist pain, swelling and tenderness in the anatomical snuff box after a fall on the outstretched hand, should be immobilised in plaster even if the X-ray is negative. A further X-ray taken out of plaster in two weeks is necessary to exclude a scaphoid fracture. The different fractures of the scaphoid are (Fig. 3.12):

    fractures of the distal pole
    fractures of the waist
    fractures of the proximal pole
    displaced fractures associated with carpal instability

* *Fractures of the distal pole* of tubercle of the scaphoid are usually uncomplicated. They will unite after immobilisation for four weeks in a scaphoid plaster.

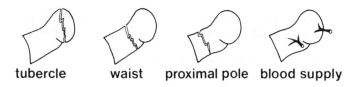

tubercle　　　**waist**　　**proximal pole**　**blood supply**

Fig. 3.12.　Fractures of the scaphoid

*** *Fractures of the waist of scaphoid*
These may be slow to unite and should be immobilised in a scaphoid plaster for eight weeks. If X-ray out of plaster shows the fracture to be still ununited, then further plaster is used for another month. If the fracture is still not united, then bone grafting of the scaphoid should be considered.

**** *Fractures of the proximal pole of the scaphoid* are treated in the same manner as those of the waist. The prognosis for union is worse. If the proximal fragment remains ununited it is probably best removed — however the prognosis for a good strong wrist is poor.

*** *Displaced fractures associated with carpal instability*
These injuries usually occur after severe accidents. The wrist may be very bruised and swollen. The patient may have other severe injuries that preclude immediate operative treatment to the wrist.

    The displaced fracture of the scaphoid is associated with a subluxation (or sometimes a complete dislocation) of the distal row of the carpus from the proximal (Fig. 3.13).

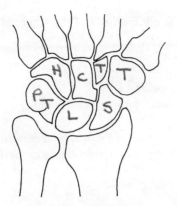

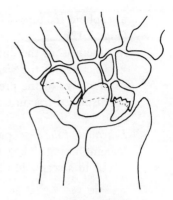

proximal & distal row
of carpal bones

trans-scaphoid perilunate
dislocation

Fig. 3.13. Carpal subluxations

These injuries are best treated by open reduction to reduce
the carpal dislocation; and to fix the scaphoid with a screw.
Fixation of the scaphoid stabilises the carpus. If early operation
is not possible the fracture should be manipulated and aligned
as best as possible until operation can be performed.

*** **Carpal subluxations**
The distal row of carpal bones (in particular the capitate)
becomes subluxed from the proximal row (in particular the
lunate and scaphoid). The subluxation may be associated
with a fracture of the scaphoid or of the radial styloid.

In some cases the distal row of the carpus is completely
dislocated from the lunate. This is known as a perilunate
dislocation (Fig. 3.13).

On occasions the distal row of carpus realigns itself with
the forearm. In realigning the distal row, the lunate becomes
squeezed out of position. This appears on the X-ray as a
'dislocated lunate'.

Carpal subluxations are often misdiagnosed. The signs are
subtle. In the A-P view there is loss of congruence of the
capitate with the scaphoid and lunate (Fig. 3.13). In the lateral
view there is a loss of alignment of the convexity of the capitate
with the concavity of the lunate (Fig. 3.14).

Scaphoid
Lunate
Triquetral
Pisiform
Hamate
Capitate
Trapezoid
Trapezium

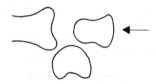

radius lunate capitate

carpal dislocation

dislocated lunate

Fig. 3.14. Mid-carpal dislocations

The median nerve may be involved in these lesions.

These injuries are difficult to manage conservatively and usually require operation.

* **Flake fractures of the carpus**
These occur fairly commonly and are seen on X-ray over the dorsum of the wrist. They require symptomatic treatment — usually a below-elbow plaster for three weeks.

*** *A fracture of the hook of the hamate* requires special X-ray views to demonstrate it. It may proceed to non-union and thus cause persistent symptoms until excised.

4 Fractures of the Wrist

** Colles' fracture
*** Smith's fracture
** Fractures of the radial styloid
*** Dislocations of the wrist
* Wrist sprains

Fractures around the wrist commonly occur through the lower end of the radius and ulna. Most unite without serious sequelae and most patients have little complaint. However, the lower end of the radius consists of cancellous bone. A fracture through this area unites with some degree of collapse. Malunion results.

These fractures also tend to be comminuted. They occur in middle-aged and elderly ladies whose bones are often osteo-porotic. These comminuted fractures almost always unite with collapse and malunion. This malunion shows itself as a shortening of the lower end of the radius and as a result the inferior radio-ulnar joint becomes subluxed and the ulnar styloid very prominent on the ulnar side of the wrist.

In any case fractures through the lower end of the radius may disrupt the inferior radio-ulnar joint. Disruption of this joint interferes with the rotational movement of the forearm bones. Patients will complain of clicking on performing this movement after fracture union. There may be limitation of rotation and pain.

In some patients the fracture line may actually extend into the wrist joint. Following union of the fracture there may be some residual stiffness of the wrist which will never restore itself to normal. It is possible that osteoarthritis will occur in a wrist after this type of fracture.

The commonest cause of a fracture of the lower end of the radius is a fall on the outstretched hand. This tends to force the hand and the distal fragment into supination relative to the forearm bones. On X-ray this will show itself as a dorsal displacement of the distal fragment and also it will be radially deviated.

A typical Colles' fracture is situated between 1 and 2 cm from the articular surface of the lower end of the radius. There is frequently an associated fracture of the ulnar styloid. The fracture is displaced dorsally and there is some impaction of the fragments and radial deviation of the distal portion. The classical deformity is that of a dinner fork.

The bones of the lower end of the wrist have a very precise relationship one to the other. The radial styloid is 1.25 cm distal to the ulnar styloid. The articular surface of the lower end of the radius is angled in a volar direction of about 10° from the vertical (Fig. 4.1).

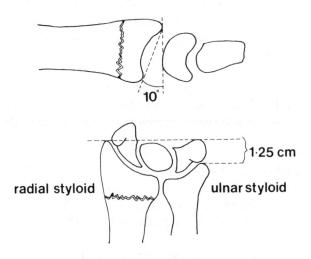

Fig. 4.1. Undisplaced Colles' fracture

All degrees of displacement of fractures of the lower end of the wrist are found and the acceptable position depends very much on the patient and the treating surgeon.

All Colles-type fractures are dorsally displaced and tend to be supinated relative to the forearm bones. Reduction involves a forced pronation and ulnar deviation movement of the distal fragment.

The reverse is known as the Smith's fracture. This tends to occur in younger people and results from much more severe violence. Smith's fractures frequently result from motorcycle injuries. On impact the motorcyclist is clutching his handle bars with his wrist in full pronation. The impact increases this pronation movement producing a fracture which is displaced in a volar direction and also is deviated radially. The distal fragment is forcibly pronated in relation to the forearm bones. Various types of Smith's fractures are described depending on the size of the distal fragment. They can be reduced by forced supination and ulnar deviation of the distal fragment on the proximal fragment.

These fractures also tend to be comminuted and heal with some collapse of the lower end of the radius. Some malunion is a common sequela.

Immediate local complications are rare. Occasionally an acute carpal tunnel syndrome can result from haematoma in the anterior compartment. Very occasionally this requires operative release.

Late onset of carpal tunnel syndrome does occur but usually resolves itself spontaneously. Every so often this syndrome is prolonged and severe enough to warrant operative decompression.

* Undisplaced Colles' fracture

A truly undisplaced Colles' fracture will have the radial styloid one centimetre distal to the ulnar styloid. The articular surface of the lower end of the radius will face 10° in a volar direction (Fig. 4.1).

An acceptable position varies with the treating doctor and depends on the age and the fitness of the patient and also on the adjudged possibilities of improving the position by manipulation.

A Colles' fracture in acceptable position should be treated initially by a dorsi-radial below-elbow plaster slab. This can be completed after a week. Plaster is retained for five weeks.

** Displaced Colles' fracture (Fig. 4.2)

A displaced Colles' fracture is reduced by manipulation under general anaesthetic. This involves the following procedures (Fig. 4.3):

the elbow is steadied by an assistant;

the fracture is disimpacted by traction and slight supination of the wrist;

the fracture is then reduced by forced and full pronation movement;

a below-elbow dorsi-radial slab is applied and moulded to apply three-point pressure:

over the proximal forearm on the radial side;

over the second metacarpal;

over the fracture site on the ulnar side and on the volar aspect.

This last can be done by moulding the plaster over the surgeon's thigh. The hand is immobilised in slight palmar flexion and full ulnar deviation.

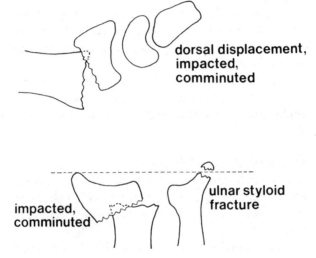

dorsal displacement, impacted, comminuted

impacted, comminuted

ulnar styloid fracture

Fig. 4.2. Displaced Colles' fracture

The following day the plaster is checked and the patient instructed as regards shoulder and finger movements.

After a week an X-ray is taken to check the position and the plaster completed. If necessary, shoulder and finger exercises are supervised by a physiotherapist.

The plaster is removed after five weeks and a full programme of exercises instituted.

A Colles' fracture has many complications for so common a lesion:

1 Shoulder stiffness;

2 Finger stiffness;

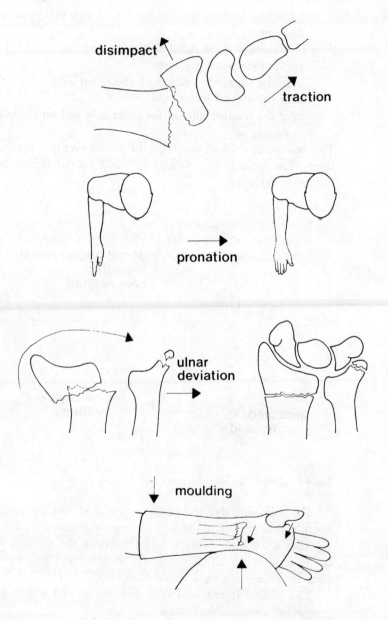

Fig. 4.3. Reduction of Colles' fracture

3 Stiffness of the wrist — particularly if the fracture extended into the joint. This stiffness would improve with exercise;

4 Malunion. The fracture is through cancellous bone of the lower end of the radius. Union almost inevitably occurs with some collapse.

The commonest deformity is shortening of the radius and this is accompanied by a prominence of the lower end of the ulna. In addition, rotation movements of the forearm may be lost and those that are retained are painful.

If severe this can be treated by excising the lower end of the ulna.

5 Carpal tunnel syndrome occurs after Colles' fracture. In the majority of patients this improves with time — occasionally operation is necessary to decompress it.

6 An attrition rupture of extensor pollicis longus is described.

*** Smith's fracture (reverse Colles' fracture)

This is a fracture through the lower end of the radius with volar displacement (Fig. 4.4). It occurs most often in young male patients due to a pronation force over the lower end of the radius.

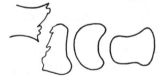

Fig. 4.4.   Smith's fracture

Various types are described depending on the shape of the fracture. One type has only a small radial fragment which splits the articular surface. This type is very unstable and behaves like a fracture subluxation of the wrist.

Smith's fractures can be reduced under general anaesthesia by traction and forced supination. In order to hold the position an above-elbow plaster is frequently necessary.

It is reasonable to operate on unstable Smith's fractures and fix them with a buttress plate.

** **Radial styloid fractures** (Fig. 4.5)

These occur frequently in young patients and involve the articular surface of the wrist joint. They are treated by four weeks immobilisation in a below-elbow plaster. Following this exercises are necessary to restore movement.

Unfortunately this fracture is frequently followed by limitation of wrist movement.

Displaced radial styloid fractures may be associated with a dislocation of the carpus or a dislocation of the wrist.

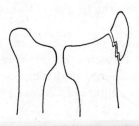

Fig. 4.5. Radial styloid fracture

*** **Wrist dislocations**

This lesion occurs occasionally and is very unstable. It is usually associated with small fractures of the lower end of the radius.

Operation is usually necessary to maintain reduction by pinning the small radial fragment in position.

* **Wrist sprains**

Injuries to the wrist are common. Many patients have a painful, swollen wrist and an X-ray reveals no fracture.

Such patients are best treated by plaster immobilisation for two or three weeks to relieve symptoms. On removing the plaster a further X-ray is taken to make sure no scaphoid fracture is missed.

In some patients the symptoms may be due to a lesion of the inferior radio-ulnar joint. These may develop chronic symptoms of pain on rotation and a clicking sensation. The treatment of these people is difficult.

WRIST FRACTURES IN CHILDREN

Juxta-epiphyseal fractures.
Fractures through the lower end of the radius well proximal to
the growth plate.

Juxta-epiphyseal fractures (Fig. 4.6)
These are usually Salter type II fractures. The distal fragment
includes a flake of metaphysis as well as the growth plate and
epiphysis.

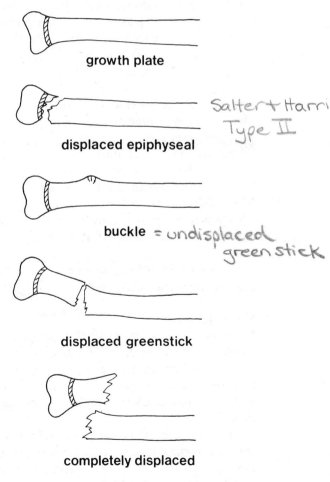

growth plate

displaced epiphyseal

Salter + Harris
Type II

buckle = undisplaced
greenstick

displaced greenstick

completely displaced

Fig. 4.6. Fractures of the lower end of the radius in children

Chapter 4

The fracture may be undisplaced (or mildly displaced), or significantly displaced. The displacement is usually dorsal but may be in a volar direction.

★ *Undisplaced juxta-epiphyseal fractures* can be treated with a below-elbow dorsal plaster slab and converted later to a complete plaster. This plaster is retained for four weeks.

★★ *Displaced juxta-epiphyseal fractures* can be reduced by manipulation under general anaesthetic. In young children remodelling of these fractures is remarkable and a considerable degree of angulation can be accepted.

Fractures with dorsal displacement should be immobilised in an above-elbow plaster slab with the wrist in pronation. Those with volar displacement should be immobilised with the wrist in supination. After a few days the position is checked by X-ray and the plaster completed.

Fractures of the lower end of the radius
These occur well proximal to the growth plate and often involve the lower end of the ulna:

★ Undisplaced buckle fractures;
★★ Greenstick fractures with dorsal or volar angulation;
★★★ Complete fractures of the radius and ulna or of the radius

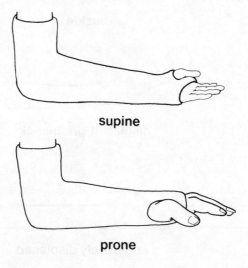

supine

prone

Fig. 4.7. Above-elbow plaster

coupled with a greenstick fracture of the ulna. These fractures are usually dorsally displaced.

* *Undisplaced buckle fractures* can be treated initially with above-elbow plaster slabs which are completed later and retained for four weeks. These fractures tend to angulate in below-elbow plasters.

** *Greenstick fractures* are reduced under general anaesthesia. Those fractures with dorsal angulation are immobilised in above-elbow plaster slabs with the hand pronated; those fractures with volar displacement have the hand in supination (Fig. 4.7). After a few days a check X-ray is taken and the plaster completed.

*** *Complete fractures* of the lower end of the radius can be difficult to reduce. Good alignment of the fractures must be obtained and maintained. Remodelling at this level in young children is good. However, rotation movement of the forearm can be permanently impaired if a significant degree of angulation is accepted. Above-elbow plaster with the wrist in the appropriate position is used.

5 Forearm Fractures

*** Fractures of both radius and ulna
** Isolated fractures of the ulna
** Isolated fractures of the radius
*** Monteggia fractures
*** Galeazzi fractures
** Forearm fractures in children

Fractures of both radius and ulna

These fractures are difficult to manage. They frequently occur in seriously ill patients with other injuries, treatment of which takes precedence. The main complications are:

1 Closed compartment syndrome. This affects the muscles of the flexor aspect of the forearm and also the median nerve. Volkmann's ischaemic contracture can be the end result. This syndrome can follow open operations on the forearm as well as closed treatment of fractures.

2 Delayed union and non-union. Fractures of the shafts of forearm bones are rather slow to unite in adults — immobilisation for twelve weeks is often necessary.

3 Malunion and loss of forearm rotation. Rotation movement occurs throughout the forearm as well as the inferior and superior radio-ulnar joints. It depends on a normal interosseous membrane and a normal relationship of the radius and ulna to it and to each other. Any degree of malunion reduces the range of forearm rotation.

It is right therefore to obtain anatomical reduction of forearm fractures by open reduction and plating.

** *Undisplaced fractures of both radius and ulna* can be treated initially by above-elbow slabs with the hand in neutral position. Later the plaster is completed. The elbow is at right angles. The plaster should be compressed in the dorsal-volar direction so that the radius and ulna are separated as much as possible. This allows the interosseous membrane to reform normally (Fig. 5.1).

*** *Displaced fractures of the radius and ulna* require anatomical

78

reduction. They are difficult to reduce by closed means and the reduction is difficult to hold in plaster.

Plates are usually used to fix the fragments. If the operation is delayed or the fracture very comminuted a cancellous bone graft can be applied at the time of plating.

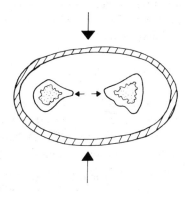

Fig. 5.1. Moulding radius and ulnar fractures

Isolated fractures of the ulna shaft
These usually occur as a result of direct violence to the forearm. They are slow to unite. An X-ray must be taken of the elbow to exclude dislocation of the head of the radius.
★★ *Undisplaced fractures of the ulna* can be treated in an above-elbow plaster for about ten weeks.
★★★ *Displaced fractures of the ulna* are probably best plated. Closed reduction is difficult and union is slow.

Isolated fractures of the shaft of the radius
These are also slow to unite. The wrist joint should always be X-rayed to exclude disruption of the inferior radio-ulnar joint.
★★ *Undisplaced fractures* should be treated in an above-elbow plaster for eight weeks.
★★★ *Displaced fractures* are probably best plated.

★★★ **Monteggia fractures**
✳ These are fractures of the upper shaft of the ulna with dislocation of the radial head. They usually occur as a result of a direct

blow on the ulnar border of the forearm. There are several variants of this fracture.

In order to diagnose the injury it is necessary to have a lateral X-ray of the elbow with the forearm at right angles to the upper arm. In this position the radial head should be in line with the radial shaft and centred on the capitellum (Fig. 5.2).

These fractures may be difficult to reduce and hold reduced. In adults they are best treated by an open operation and plating of the ulnar shaft fracture.

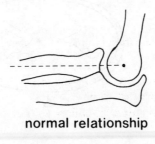

normal relationship

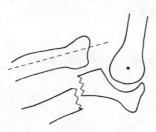

Fig. 5.2.   Monteggia fracture dislocation

*** **Galleazzi fractures**
These are fractures of the lower third of the shaft of the radius with disruption of the inferior radio-ulnar joint (Fig. 5.3). In order to diagnose them an A-P X-ray centred on the wrist joint is necessary.

These fractures are unstable. They are best treated by open reduction and plating of the fractured radius.

Forearm fractures in children
* Undisplaced fractures of one or both bones

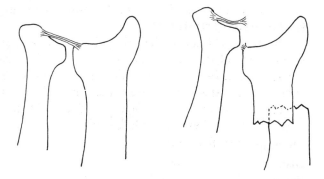

Fig. 5.3. Galleazzi fracture

★★ Greenstick fractures with angulation
★★★ Complete fractures of both bones
★★★ Monteggia fractures in children

★ *Undisplaced fractures* of one or both bones can be simply immobilised in an above-elbow plaster with the hand in neutral position.

★★ *Angulated greenstick fractures* require manipulation under general anaesthesia. The arm is immobilised in above-elbow slabs with the hand in appropriate position. After a few days the plaster is completed and the position checked by X-ray.

Plaster should be retained for four to six weeks depending on the age of the child.

★★★ *Complete fractures of both bones* are difficult to reduce and hold reduced. A trial manipulation under general anaesthesia should be tried and a carefully moulded plaster applied.

However, if this is unsuccessful or the fracture becomes displaced in plaster these fractures are better plated.

★★★ *Monteggia fractures in children* can be reduced by manipulation and the reduction held in plaster. However, this may fail or the injury may become redisplaced in which case open reduction is necessary.

6 Elbow Injuries

ELBOW INJURIES IN ADULTS

* The contused elbow
** Dislocations of the elbow
** Fractures of the radial head
*** Fractures of the olecranon
* Flake fractures of the coronoid
*** Fractures of the capitellum
*** T-shaped fractures of the humerus

* The contused elbow

Patients commonly present after injury with a bruised, swollen, painful elbow. X-ray (including oblique views) should be taken to exclude fracture. The signs of fracture are often subtle such as the 'fat pad' sign.

These injuries are best treated by a week's rest in a posterior plaster slab and sling. This is followed by graduated exercises.

** Postero-lateral dislocations of the elbow

This is the usual type of dislocation of the elbow. It is associated with disruption of the medial ligament. The medial ligament of the elbow is attached to the medial epicondyle — this may be avulsed in association with the dislocation. On occasions it may become stuck in the joint and hinder reduction of the dislocation.

A fractured coronoid is also associated with a dislocated elbow.

A postero-lateral dislocation can be difficult to reduce. A general anaesthetic with muscle relaxation is necessary. Having reduced the dislocation the elbow is immobilised in a posterior plaster slab and sling. The patient is best admitted to hospital overnight to check for complications.

Immobilisation is continued for three weeks and then very gentle graduated active exercises are started. It may take months for the patient to regain full elbow movements.

Complications of a dislocated elbow
1 Associated fractures — of medial epicondyle or coronoid. These may become implanted in the joint and impede reduction. Open reduction is then necessary.
2 Vascular complications. The brachial artery may be contused or torn.
3 Nerve lesions. Usually the ulnar nerve is involved. However, the median nerve can also be damaged.
4 Stiffness of the elbow. The joint is usually stiff for weeks or months following dislocation. Recovery is gradual with gentle active exercises. If movements are forced myositis ossificans can occur.
5 Recurrence of dislocation. This is described particularly in dislocations associated with fracture.

Other types of dislocation
Medial, lateral of even anterior dislocation.
Isolated dislocation of the radial head or of the ulna.
Dislocation of radial head associated with Monteggia fractures.

Fractures of the head of the radius (Fig. 6.1)
These occur particularly in adults after a fall on the outstretched hand. The radial head is impacted onto the capitellum and fractures. Sometimes the capitellum is damaged as well.

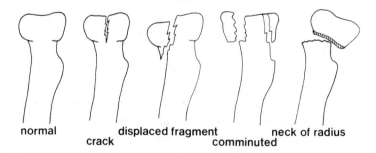

normal   displaced fragment   neck of radius
     crack   comminuted

Fig. 6.1. Fractures of the radial head

* *Minimally displaced fractures of the radial head*
These are small crack fractures with minimal displacement.

Chapter 6

They are often painful and the elbow is swollen with a haem-arthrosis.

They are best treated by immobilisation with a plaster back slab and sling. After two weeks the plaster is removed and the patient starts exercising with a loop sling.

*** *Displaced fractures of the radial head*
These include fractures:

> with a significant step in the articular surface;
> where more than one-third of the articular surface is dam-aged;
> where there are loose fracture fragments in the joint.

These fractures should be treated by operation. The radial head is excised and loose fragments removed.

Best results are obtained if the operation is performed soon after injury. Nearly a full range of elbow joint motion results although the arm does feel somewhat weaker afterwards.

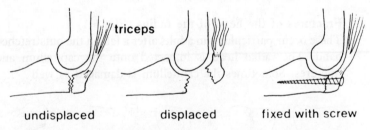

undisplaced   displaced   fixed with screw

Fig. 6.2.   Fractures of the olecranon

Fractures of the olecranon (Fig. 6.2)
Fractures of the olecranon may be widely separated by the pull of the triceps muscle. These may be reduced by extending the elbow. However, immobilisation in this position is cumber-some and the resulting stiffness difficult to overcome. Displaced fractures of the olecranon are best firmly fixed at operation.

* *Undiplaced fractures of the olecranon* can be immobilised with a posterior plaster slab with the elbow at right angles. After three weeks this is removed and active exercises started.
*** *Displaced fractures* are best treated by open reduction and the fracture fixed with a screw or tension band wiring (Fig. 6.2).

Some fractures in the elderly have a very small proximal fragment. This can be excised and the triceps expansion sewn directly onto the ulna.

**** *Fractures of the olecranon with dislocation of the radial head*
These are a type of Monteggia fracture. They are very unstable.

They may be seen after road traffic accidents and can be severely compound injuries. They may present a very difficult problem as the patients may have severe general injuries. The repair of skin and soft tissues around the elbow takes precedence over the management of this particular fracture.

Ideally the fracture of the olecranon should be firmly fixed and the head of the radius reduced.

*** **Fractures of the capitellum**
These are seen occasionally after a fall on the outstretched hand. They may be associated with fractures of the radial head.

When seen they are usually significantly displaced. If the fragments are small they are best excised. If the fragments are large they can be reduced and fixed with pins.

T-shaped fractures of the humerus (Fig. 6.3)
These occur in adults. The fracture is comminuted passing vertically from the articular surface to the supracondylar region — a transverse extension completes the T. All degrees of displacement are seen, from no displacement to a grossly displaced comminuted fracture with associated disruption of the elbow joint.

As the fracture passes into the joint the main complications are of joint stiffness and the possibility of degenerative changes occurring at a later date.

** *Undisplaced T-shaped fractures*
These can be treated with a posterior plaster slab and a sling for one or two weeks to allow swelling to subside. Then gradual active exercises are started.

**** *Displaced T-shaped fractures*
These are very difficult to treat and patients are often left with very limited flexion and extension movements.

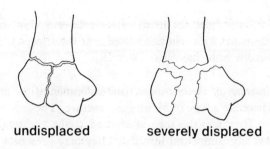

undisplaced   **severely displaced**

Fig. 6.3.   T-shaped fracture of the lower end of the humerus

If the displacement is slight it is best to treat these fractures with a posterior plaster slab for one or two weeks followed by active exercises.

If the displacement is marked the fracture fragments are often comminuted and the articular surface extensively damaged. Gentle manipulation under anaesthetic may mould the fragments into better position — early mobilisation is then undertaken.

A better X-ray appearance is obtained by operation. However the elbow tends to become so stiff that the function is not improved.

ELBOW FRACTURES IN CHILDREN

*** Supracondylar fractures
*** Lateral condyle fractures
 ** Medial epicondyle fractures
  * Radial neck fractures
 ** Olecranon fractures
  * Pulled elbow

Fractures about the elbow in children are different from those of adults. They may be difficult to diagnose from X-rays. Ossification is incomplete in children and there are numerous ossification centres about the elbow. It can be helpful to:

X-ray the normal elbow for comparison;
take extra oblique views of the elbow;
look for soft tissue abnormalities such as the fat pad sign.

Supracondylar fractures of the humerus (Fig. 6.4)
These occur in children after a fall on the outstretched arm
usually with the elbow extended.

** *Undisplaced fractures* occur and can be easily treated with a
posterior plaster slab for two weeks followed by gradual mobilisation.

*** *Displaced fractures* are usually displaced posteriorly with associated varus rotation of the distal fragment. (An anterior displaced
supracondylar fracture sometimes occurs.)

The patient presents with the arm held extended. Gross
swelling occurs rapidly. Because of the swelling a manipulation
must be performed soon. If the patient presents late, it is best
to treat the fracture with traction and perform a manipulation a
few days later when the swelling has subsided.

After reduction the elbow is held in the flexed position to
allow the triceps to maintain the fragments in alignment. This
can be maintained with a collar and cuff — a posterior plaster
slab is usually more acceptable. Operative fixation can be obtained using percutaneous pin fixation.

Complications of supracondylar fractures are numerous.

Vascular problems occur commonly and if not treated immediately a Volkmann's ischaemic contracture may supervene.

There may be damage to the brachial artery at the fracture
site. This damage may be a complete division but is usually a
contusion with disruption of the intima, or arterial spasm.

A closed compartment syndrome may occur affecting the
anterior flexor compartment of the forearm. This is made worse
by flexing the forearm on reducing the fracture.

The signs of impending vascular problems are:
pain — particularly on extending the fingers;
pallour or dusky discolouration of fingers;
loss of the radial pulse;
loss of sensation in the hand.
Treatment:
gradually release the flexed elbow;
operative intervention:
to divide fascia,
expose artery and repair if necessary,
internally fix the fracture.

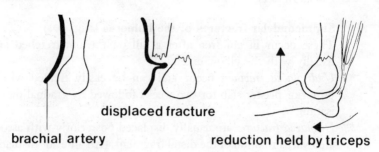

displaced fracture

brachial artery   reduction held by triceps

Fig. 6.4. Supracondylar fracture of the humerus

A Volkmann's contracture results from an ellipsoidal infarct of the muscles of the flexor compartment of the forearm. The dead muscles are replaced by fibrous tissue. This contracts and a flexion contracture of the wrist and fingers results.

The median nerve is also damaged and the greater part of the hand is anaesthetic.

A patient with a fully developed Volkmann's contracture has a very severe disability and presents as an almost impossible reconstruction problem.

Other complications:

Nerve injuries. The median nerve is most commonly damaged but the ulnar and radial nerves may be involved.

Malunion:

Cubitus varus results if rotation is not corrected.

A gunstock deformity shows hyperextension of the elbow as well as varus deformity. This follows incomplete reduction.

Elbow stiffness — this gradually resolves almost entirely. The patient (and his parents) are advised of this and only very gradual and gentle active exercises are allowed.

Myositis ossificans — arises as calcification of an organising haematoma. It was found more frequently after intensive passive physiotherapy. This is contra-indicated for elbow injuries. The treatment of this condition is rest followed by very gentle active exercises.

*** **Lateral condyle fractures of the humerus** (Fig. 6.5)

These fractures occur in young children (*aet.* 3−5 years) after a fall. The fracture involves the capitellum and the adjacent metaphysis. The fracture line passes through the growth plate and is classified as Salter type 4 lesion.

The fracture fragment is pulled away from the humerus by the extensor muscles of the forearm. This fracture requires accurate reduction otherwise arrest of growth occurs. This causes a gradually increasing cubitus valgus deformity and a tardy ulnar nerve palsy occurs as the nerve becomes stretched.

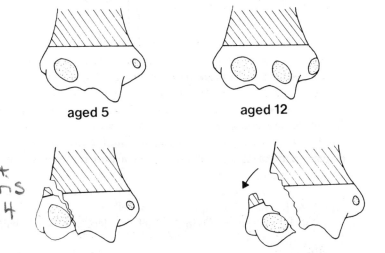

aged 5   **aged 12**

Fig. 6.5. Epiphyses of the lower end of the humerus. Displaced fracture of the lateral condyle

Undisplaced lateral condyle fractures are immobilised with a posterior plaster slab and a sling for some three weeks.

Displaced fractures require open reduction and fixation of the fragments with pins.

Fractures of the medial epicondyle (Fig. 6.6)
These are avulsion fractures which occur in older children. They may be associated with an elbow dislocation. The epicondyle fragment may be trapped inside the joint preventing reduction. A transient ulnar nerve lesion may be associated with the fracture.

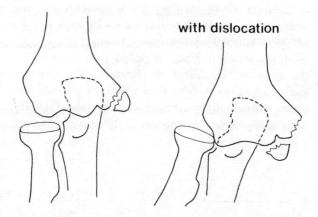

Fig. 6.6. Fractures of the medial epicondyle

* *Uncomplicated medial epicondyle fractures* can be treated by immobilisation with a plaster slab and a sling for two weeks. The displacement of the epicondyle is not a problem and a quite adequate fibrous union will occur.

*** *A complicated medial epicondyle fracture* usually requires operation. A fragment entrapped in the elbow joint should be removed by operation. Fixing it back in place with a pin will stabilise the elbow.

A fracture complicated by an ulnar nerve lesion is also best explored. The nerve can be transposed and the fragment pinned back in position.

Fractures of the radial neck (see Fig. 6.1)
These occur as a result of a fall on an outstretched arm. The radial head should never be excised in children no matter how severe the fracture. It is an actively growing centre and a deformity of the forearm will result after excision.

** *Displaced fractures* with an angulation in excess of 45° can be manipulated and the fracture reduced.

Occasionally the head is completely separated and then it should be replaced at open reduction.

Fractures of the olecranon
* *An undisplaced fracture* can be treated in flexion with a plaster slab.

** *A displaced fracture* requires reduction and can be held in extension in plaster. It is also possible to fix it with pins at operation. These pins should be removed soon after the reduction.

* **Pulled elbow**
This term is applied to a subluxation of the radial head from the annular ligament. The common cause is the parent (or guardian) yanking the child by one arm. The patient complains of pain in the elbow on movement. There may be tenderness and swelling. X-ray will show no lesion.

Treatment involves traction of the slightly flexed elbow followed by supination. The elbow should be immobilised in a collar and cuff overnight and the patient reviewed next day to confirm the cure.

** 7 Fractures of the Shaft of the Humerus

There is a spectrum of severity of these fractures. It extends from undisplaced spiral fractures to grossly comminuted high-energy fractures associated with soft tissue injury in patients with other severe injuries (Fig. 7.1). Complications include:

Radial nerve injury — this produces a wrist or finger drop. The loss of sensation is minimal and confined to a small area on the radial side of the hand.

Median and ulnar injuries also occur.

Arterial injuries are rare.

Shoulder stiffness is common and persistent.

Delayed and non-union are fairly common — particularly so in comminuted high-energy fractures after road traffic accidents.

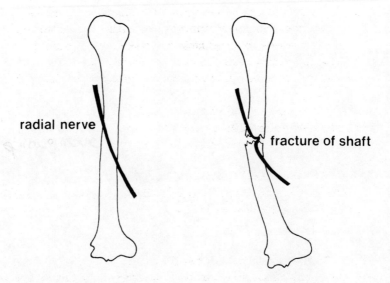

Fig. 7.1. Humerus and radial nerve

Management

Both displaced and undisplaced fractures can be adequately controlled by a U-slab plaster. This extends from the acromion around the lateral side of the arm, and thence up the inner side to the axilla. This is applied with the patient sitting and the arm hanging pendent and supported by an assistant. The fracture is aligned by gravity.

A collar cuff is applied and the arm bound to the side. After a few days the bandage can be discarded and replaced by a well-fitting T-shirt. The U-slab requires tightening over six weeks. Following this the arm can be mobilised from a sling (Fig. 7.2).

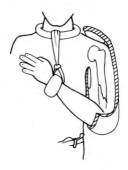

Fig. 7.2. Hanging-U POP

Patients with displaced fracture, particularly if complicated by a nerve lesion, can be treated by open reduction. They are best fixed with a plate supplemented by a cancellous bone graft.

When the radial nerve is injured the lesion is usually either a neuropraxia or an axonotmesis. It will therefore probably recover in the course of time. The results of radial nerve suture are poor in adults. The wrist and finger drop are usually treated by tendon transfer if there is no recovery.

8 Shoulder Injuries

** Dislocations of the shoulder
*** Fracture-dislocations
** Fractures of the surgical neck
*** Fractures of the greater tuberosity
* Growth plate fractures of the upper end of the humerus in children

The upper end of the humerus can be considered as consisting of four portions (Fig. 8.1a):

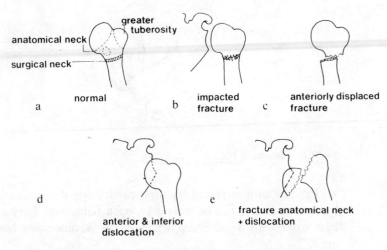

Fig. 8.1. Injuries to the neck of the humerus

1 The head of the humerus which articulates with the glenoid of the scapula. It is separated from the rest of the upper end of the humerus by the anatomical neck.
2 The greater tuberosity to which the supraspinatus and infraspinatus are attached.
3 The lesser tuberosity to which the subscapularis is attached. It is separated from the greater tuberosity by the bicipital groove.

94

4 The surgical neck separates these three structures from the proximal shaft of the humerus. The main muscles, pectoralis major, latissimus dorsi, and deltoid are attached distal to the surgical neck.

Dislocations
** *Anterior dislocation of the shoulder*

This occurs commonly in adults as a result of a variety of mechanisms.

The patient presents with a painful immobile shoulder and may give a history of previous dislocations. The contour of the shoulder is altered — being flattened — and the humerus held away from the side (Fig. 8.2).

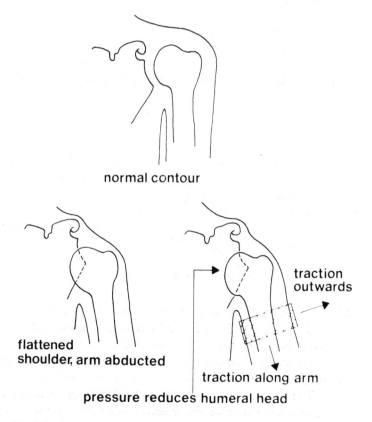

normal contour

flattened shoulder, arm abducted

traction outwards

traction along arm

pressure reduces humeral head

Fig. 8.2. Reduction of a dislocated shoulder

X-rays should always be taken before attempting reduction (unless the patient has a definite history of recurrent dislocation). Fractures are often associated with the dislocation.

The dislocation is best reduced in hospital under general anaesthesia with X-ray control.

The best method of reduction is by a modified Hippocratic method. Traction is exerted on the arm by an assistant and it is partly abducted. The arm is then internally rotated and the surgeon presses the head into the glenoid by direct backward pressure (Fig. 8.2).

Following reduction, the shoulder is immobilised with a sling worn under the clothes for three weeks. This allows the shoulder capsule time to heal and reduces the likelihood of recurrent dislocation.

Complications

1 Axillary nerve palsy — there is no contraction of the deltoid. There is also an area of hypo-aesthesia over the outer upper arm in the distribution of the lateral cutaneous nerve of the upper arm.

2 Brachial plexus palsy — this is uncommon and is usually a distal incomplete lesion with a good prognosis for eventual recovery.

3 Damage to the axillary artery has been described. It is a danger when reducing a long-standing dislocation.

4 Associated fracture of greater tuberosity or anatomical neck of the humerus

5 Shoulder stiffness — this is found particularly in the elderly in whom there is frequently a rotator cuff tear. It is also marked after fracture dislocations.

6 Recurrence of dislocation is common.

*** *Subluxio-erecta dislocation of the shoulder*
This is a rare dislocation. The head of the humerus is impacted below the glenoid.

The patient presents with the arm in fixed abduction above the head. The lesion is frequently associated with a rotator cuff lesion. Reduction is urgent as the axillary vessels and brachial plexus are liable to be compressed.

*** *Posterior dislocation of the shoulder*
This is uncommon and difficult to diagnose. It occurs after severe trauma or after epileptic fits or electric shocks.

The patient should be examined from above and it will be seen (and felt) that the head of the humerus is not in its normal position (Fig. 8.3). The arm tends to be held in internal rotation and there is loss of external rotation.

The X-ray signs are subtle. There is an abnormality detectable on A-P X-ray. An axial lateral X-ray will demonstrate the dislocation unequivocally, it may be necessary to anaesthetise the patient to show this.

Reduction of the dislocation is not difficult but it tends to redislocate very easily.

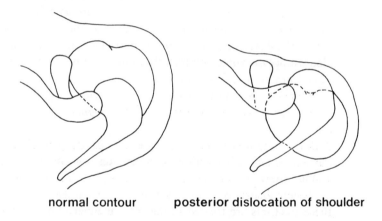

normal contour   posterior dislocation of shoulder

Fig. 8.3. Shoulder from above

Fracture-dislocation of the shoulder
** *Associated with fractures of the greater tuberosity.* The shoulder should be reduced. If the fracture of the greater tuberosity then lies in reasonable alignment the patient can be treated as for an uncomplicated dislocation.

However, if the fracture becomes displaced up under the acromion it requires open reduction and fixation with a screw.

Chapter 8

**** *Associated with fractures of the anatomical neck* (Fig. 8.3). This is a severe injury to the shoulder. It may occur in old and debilitated people. If indicated the dislocation is reduced by operation. Unfortunately the articular portion will probably undergo avascular necrosis as it has lost its blood supply.

A few patients with this lesion benefit from a prosthetic replacement for the humeral head.

*** *Associated with fracture of the surgical neck.* These fractures also probably require open reduction but the prognosis for survival of the head is good.

Fractures of the surgical neck

** *Impacted fractures of the surgical neck* (Fig. 8.1d)
These are common injuries in elderly and middle-aged women after a fall on the outstretched arm. They are associated with considerable pain, bruising, and swelling of the shoulder.

As the fracture fragments are impacted together and the blood supply is good, the fracture unites readily. However, the gleno-humeral joint becomes stiff.

They can be simply treated by a broad arm sling under the clothes for a week or ten days. Following this intensive exercises are prescribed.

The prognosis for useful movement in the gleno-humeral joint is poor. The patient compensates by increasing her scapulo-thoracic range.

When associated with fractures of the greater tuberosity these fractures are treated in the same manner. The prognosis for useful gleno-humeral movement after injury is worse.

*** *Displaced fractures of the surgical neck* (Fig. 8.1c)
These occur occasionally in elderly people and in younger patients after road traffic accidents.

The distal fragment (the proximal humeral shaft) is usually displaced anteriorly towards the axillary vessels and the brachial plexus. Fortunately injury to these structures is uncommon.

These fractures are best reduced under general anaesthesia monitored by an image intensifier. It is usually possible to hitch the fracture fragments into a stable position. The fracture can then be treated with a sling under the clothes for three weeks before mobilising.

If the fracture cannot be reduced by manipulation it can be reduced by open operation and fixed with pins and figure-of-eight wiring.

*** **Fractures of the greater tuberosity**
These are often associated with other injuries such as fractures of the surgical neck and dislocations.

Undisplaced fractures can be treated as impacted fractures of the surgical neck of the humerus.

Displaced fractures are best managed by open operation to reduce the fracture and fix it with a screw.

Growth plate fractures of the upper end of the humerus in children
* *Undisplaced fractures* are very common. They can be treated with a sling under the clothes for a week and then a sling outside the clothes for a further two or three weeks. They rapidly return to normal.

*** *Displaced fractures* are often associated with other severe injuries — there may be gross displacement.

Fortunately the fracture is close to the growth plate and remodels dramatically. It never requires reduction.

These children can be treated with a sling under their clothes for three weeks. They can exercise the shoulder from the sling for the next three weeks.

9 Shoulder Girdle Injuries

*** Fractures of the scapula
* Fractures of the clavicle
** Acromio-clavicular subluxations and dislocations
*** Sterno-clavicular dislocations

Fractures of the scapula

*** *Fractures of the blade of the scapula*
The scapula is covered by muscle and is well protected from trauma. It requires severe violence to fracture it.

These fractures are often associated with other injuries — in particular fractures of the underlying ribs and damage to lungs and pleura. There is often considerable bleeding from contused muscle and hypovolaemic shock may result.

Fractures of the blade of the scapula can be treated symptomatically with a sling for two weeks followed by mobilising exercises. However, it is wise to admit such patients to hospital for a day or two for observation to exclude the above complications.

** *Fractures of the neck of the scapula* are seen occasionally. They may be displaced. Symptomatic treatment with a sling is all that is necessary.

** *Fractures of the glenoid* occur and may be associated with a shoulder dislocation. These also can be treated with a sling. Occasionally the glenoid can be split by the fracture, in which case it is necessary to operate and reconstitute the glenoid in order to restore stability to the shoulder joint.

** *Fractures of the acromion and coracoid* are also seen as isolated injuries. They may also be found in combination with other shoulder fractures. Symptomatic treatment with a sling followed by mobilising exercises is all that is necessary.

Fractures of the clavicle (Fig. 9.1)
These are common fractures resulting from a fall on the outstretched arm.

100

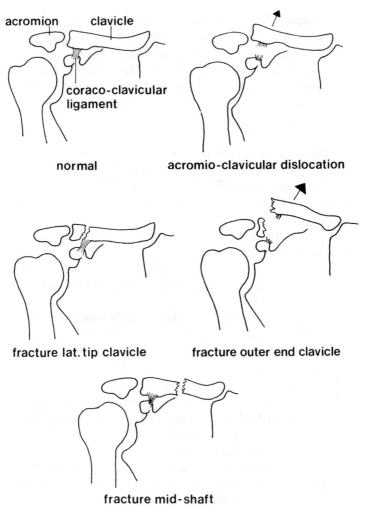

Fig. 9.1.   Injuries of the clavicle, acromio-clavicular joint

They may also be found after severe injuries such as road traffic accidents. These patients may have associated chest injuries. They may also have badly displaced and comminuted fractures with involvement of brachial plexus or subclavian vessels.

Fractures of the clavicle shaft usually unite readily. An

unsightly bulge can occur at the fracture site. This usually remodels satisfactorily in the course of a year or eighteen months. Occasionally these fractures take a long time to unite. Every so often non-union occurs. An ununited clavicle usually causes significant symptoms and should be operated on. The non-union is fixed with an intramedullary pin and a cancellous bone graft is applied.

Fractures midshaft of clavicle
* *An undisplaced or slightly displaced fracture of the clavicle* can be adequately immobilised in a broad arm sling worn under the clothes for two weeks. Exercises can then be prescribed from a sling outside the clothes. Most such patients are fit to return to work in six weeks.
** *A displaced or comminuted fracture* can be treated with a figure-of-eight bandage or similar appliance. This tends to brace back the shoulders and re-align the clavicle. The shoulder is supported by a broad arm sling worn under the clothes.

After two weeks the bandage can be discarded. After four weeks mobilising exercises are started from the sling.

Fracture of the outer end of the clavicle
* *Fracture of the lateral tip* (Fig. 9.1). The main fragment of the clavicle is fixed down by the coraco-clavicular ligament and there is little displacement. The fracture can be adequately treated with a broad arm sling.
*** *Fracture of the lateral third* (Fig. 9.1). The fracture may be associated with disruption of the coraco-clavicular ligament. There may be marked displacement of the proximal fragment as it is no longer held in position.

Such fractures are best operated on and fixed with an intramedullary pin.

* *Fractures of the clavicle in children*
These are very common fractures indeed. Sometimes they are difficult to detect on X-ray and special views should be taken. They unite readily and remodelling of the fracture site is eventually perfect.

They are best managed by a broad arm sling worn under the clothes for two weeks. This is followed by a sling outside the clothes for two weeks — by which time the shoulder is usually restored to normal.

Displaced and comminuted fractures can be treated with a figure-of-eight bandage as well as a broad arm sling.

*** **Acromio-clavicular joint subluxations and dislocations** (Fig. 9.1)
The acromio-clavicular joint is surrounded by capsular ligaments. However the clavicle is firmly attached to the coracoid of the scapula by strong coraco-clavicular ligaments.

An injury to the point of the shoulder damages the capsular ligament and allows a subluxation of the acromio-clavicular joint to occur. If the coraco-clavicular ligament is also disrupted a dislocation results — the outer end of the clavicle is obvious as a bony prominence.

The clavicle is attached at its medial end to the sternum — an injury to the acromio-clavicular joint can be associated with a lesion of the sterno-clavicular joint.

An acromio-clavicular dislocation can also be but a part of a more serious injury affecting the chest wall.

* *An acromio-clavicular subluxation* can be treated symptomatically with a broad arm sling. There may well be a slight residual prominence but this is usually asymptomatic.

*** *An acromio-clavicular dislocation* is difficult to hold reduced by any conservative method.

The deformity can be ignored. The dislocation is treated with a sling and early mobilising exercises. The prominence of the outer end of the clavicle remains but gradually becomes less pronounced and is not usually painful. If it does cause symptoms the outer end of the clavicle can be resected.

This treatment is appropriate for more elderly patients and for those who wish to avoid an operation.

In young, fit and athletic patients it is probably best to perform an open reduction. The clavicle can be fixed to the coracoid with a screw. Alternatively the acromio-clavicular joint can be fixed with a pin. In any case the fixation device must be removed in three months otherwise it will fret and break.

*** **Sterno-clavicular dislocations**
These occur as a result of compression across the shoulders

103

being transmitted along the clavicle to the sterno-clavicular joint. They may be associated with other severe injuries — especially chest injuries. An anterior dislocation usually results. A posterior dislocation can result directly from violence over the inner end of the clavicle.

These lesions are difficult to diagnose on X-ray and are best diagnosed clinically.

An anterior sterno-clavicular dislocation will manifest as a prominence of the medial end of the clavicle associated with bruising and swelling. It can be reduced but tends to redislocate. It is best to accept the deformity. In time it becomes less obvious and causes little functional disability.

In some patients the joint persistently dislocates and relocates. This causes painful symptoms. This recurrent dislocation can be repaired by operation.

A posterior sterno-clavicular dislocation is less common. Cases are described with pressure symptoms involving the great vessels, trachea or oesophagus.

These dislocations can usually be reduced under general anaesthesia with relaxation. They often slip into place on performing the manoeuvre of intubating the patient. Very occasionally open reduction is required.

10 Injuries of the Cervical Spine

*** Atlanto-axial dislocations
*** Fractures of the arch of the atlas
*** Fractures of the odontoid
*** Hangman's fracture
*** Bifacet dislocations of cervical spine
*** Unifacet dislocations of cervical spine
*** Compression fractures of vertebral bodies
*** Hyperextension injuries

These can be difficult to diagnose and to manage. The patient himself is ever aware of the complication of tetraplegia (see p. 121). Most fractures and also most dislocations of the cervical spine do not have any neurological problems. Only the more severely displaced or unstable lesions are so complicated. The complications of cervical spine injury are:
Instability
Neurological damage
Misdiagnosis

INSTABILITY

The spine is stable when there is no tendency for further displacement to occur after injury.

The spine is unstable when it displaces unless properly immobilised. Such displacement not only results in deformity, it may precipitate neurological complications. In order to prevent further damage care must be taken in moving patients with spinal injury. They should be carried in 'one straight piece' with the spine extended at the fracture. Three persons are required to lift and one to supervise. If the patient has a neck injury the supervisor should hold the head, keeping the neck in extension.

Instability can be classified as:

1 *Immediate* — following directly after injury. Dislocations of the cervical spine cause disruption of the posterior elements

105

at the level affected, the superspinous and the interspinous ligaments and the facet joints. Such lesions are easy to reduce but redisplace as easily.

Careful reduction and immobilisation of the cervical spine is necessary to allow the posterior structures to heal and allow stability. Such immobilisation can be obtained by the use of skull traction with the patient lying flat on a turning bed or operative reduction and fusion of the affected segment.

2 *Late*. Late instability can result from imperfect healing of a fracture dislocation. It can also result following a comminuted fracture of a vertebral body. A 'burst' fracture may have a large teardrop fragment anteriorly — such a fracture is particularly liable to heal with collapse of the vertebral body. A kyphotic deformity of the spine results which may of itself cause neurological symptoms (see Fig. 10.7).

NEUROLOGICAL DAMAGE

Neurological damage involves not only the spinal cord but also the nerve roots at the level of the injury.

High cervical lesions can involve the higher centres. The patient may die. More distal lesions damage the cord completely or incompletely. Most neurological damage occurs at the time of injury and is irreversible.

It is generally recognised that a patient rendered totally tetraplegic after injury will show no worthwhile recovery. Total tetraplegia means not only complete motor and sensory loss below the level of the lesion but also loss of nerve supply to bladder and anus. If any portion is spared then there is a possibility of recovery. Various syndromes of incomplete tetraplegia are described.

All patients with significant neck injury should be examined for neurological deficit as thoroughly as possible. This examination should be repeated to monitor their neurological state.

If the causative lesion is a dislocation this should be reduced as soon as possible. If there is evidence of bone and disc fragments pressing on the cord anteriorly there is good evidence for removing them. After such an exploratory operation the cervical spine should be fused to help stabilize it. However there is no evidence that these procedures actually induce recovery. An exploratory laminectomy (from the back) is almost always contra-indicated in neck injuries as it makes the instability so much worse.

The vertebral canal is wide in the cervical region. It is narrowed and more rigid in people with cervical spondylosis and ankylosing spondylitis. These patients in particular are liable to neurological complications after hyperextension injury. Such injury rarely causes neurological problems in a patient with a previously normal mobile spine.

MISDIAGNOSIS

Head injuries are associated with injuries of the cervical spine. Any patient with a significant head injury (especially if rendered unconscious) must be examined and X-rayed to exclude a neck lesion.

Cervical spine injuries may be difficult to diagnose on X-ray. Special views have to be taken. The CAT scanner adds a third diagnostic dimension.

In particular lesions between C6−7 and between C7−T1 are frequently missed. Lateral X-rays may not show these levels in thick-necked patients — particularly if there is spasm of the neck muscles.

C1   C2
*** **Atlanto-axial dislocations**
These are uncommon as a direct result of trauma. However, they are seen in association with other pathology.

Patients with rheumatoid arthritis are liable to develop increased laxity and dislocation at this level — as at other levels in the cervical spine.

Children with infections in the retropharyngeal region are likely to develop atlanto-axial dislocations. These will heal, if the neck is immobilised, after resolution of the original infection.

*** **Fractures of the arch of the atlas** (Fig. 10.1) C1
These occur occasionally after compression injuries. The arch of the atlas is fractured and the fragments spread apart. The lesion is potentially unstable.

These patients are best treated by immobilisation on a turning bed using skull traction (see Fig. 2.8). After six or eight

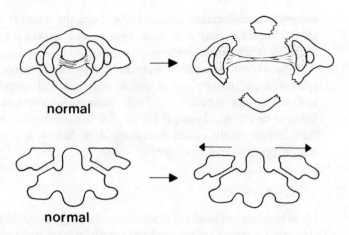

normal

normal

Fig. 10.1. Fracture of the atlas

minerva plaster

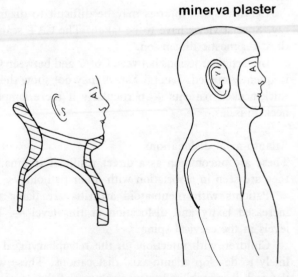

Fig. 10.2. Cervical brace and minerva plaster

weeks a minerva plaster or cervical brace can be applied (Fig. 10.2). This is worn until the fracture is united.

*** **Fractures of the odontoid** (Fig. 10.3) C2
These occur either through the isthmus or at the base of the odontoid. The patient complains of neck pain and tends to

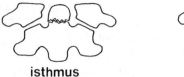 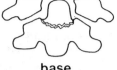

isthmus   base

Fig. 10.3. Odontoid fractures

support his head in his hands as it feels unstable. There are usually no neurological signs if the patient survives.

The fracture can be seen on a lateral X-ray of the upper cervical spine. A through-mouth A-P view must be taken.

These fractures are unstable. The patient is treated initially on a turning bed with skull traction. Later a minerva plaster or cervical brace can be applied. A halobrace can be used; this provides more rigid fixation and allows the patient to be mobilised more rapidly.

Unfortunately fractures through the isthmus tend not to unite. Fibrous union of the odontoid results, which may cause late instability. There is a good case for fusion of these un-united fractures from atlas to axis if the patients general condition warrants it.

*** **Hangman's fracture** (Fig. 10.4)

This is a fracture through the pedicle and lamina of axis with instability between the axis and the third cervical vertebra.

Road traffic accidents are now the commonest cause of this lesion. There are usually no neurological symptoms in patients who survive. Judicial hanging produced a similar lesion but with distraction of the fragments.

The fractures are unstable and require treatment on a turning bed and a collar (traction may distract the fracture making it more unstable). After six or eight weeks, a minerva plaster or cervical brace can be worn. These fractures usually unite satisfactorily.

*** **Bifacet dislocations of the cervical spine** (Fig. 10.5)

These occur as a result of road traffic accidents or sports injuries. They are probably due to a forced flexion mechanism. They often cause tetraplegia.

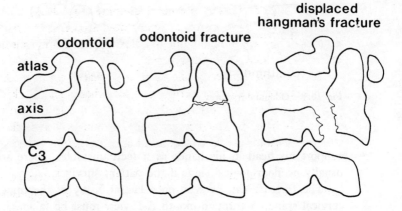

Fig. 10.4. Odontoid fractures

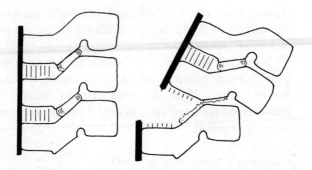

Fig. 10.5. Bifacet dislocation of the vertebrae

The patients are treated by traction on a turning bed and the dislocation gradually reduced (see Fig. 2.8). If the dislocation cannot be reduced by traction then open reduction is necessary. The spine is fixed with wire and grafted.

In most cases a satisfactory reduction can be obtained by traction and immobilisation is continued for two months. Following this a minerva plaster is applied and retained for a further two or three months until the dislocation is stabilised (Fig. 10.3).

Unfortunately after this type of dislocation the posterior ligament complex does not always heal adequately. The cervical spine then requires stabilisation by spinal fusion.

*** **Unifacet dislocations of the cervical spine** (Fig. 10.6)
These also occur as a result of road traffic accidents or sports injuries. They are probably due to a flexion and rotation mechanism. They may cause tetraplegia.

In these patients only one facet is displaced and the displacement forward of one vertebra on the other is less marked.

The patients are treated with traction on a turning bed to try and reduce the fracture gradually. Frequently a unifacet dislocation cannot be so reduced and open reduction is necessary. The spine is fused at the same time.

If the dislocation can be reduced by traction it is treated as for bifacet dislocation. Fortunately the posterior complex of ligaments heals better in unifacet dislocations and late instability is not so much of a problem.

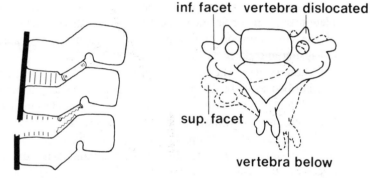

inf. facet   vertebra dislocated

sup. facet

vertebra below

Fig. 10.6. Unifacet dislocation of the vertebrae

Compression fractures
These result from a vertical compression mechanism and occur from a variety of injuries. The posterior ligament complex is usually intact but instability can result if the fracture of the vertebral body is very comminuted.

*** *A wedge compression fracture* occurs although less frequently than in the dorsal spine (Fig. 10.7a).

These fractures can be treated simply with a firm collar for a few weeks.

*** *A bursting fracture* is a more severe injury. A CAT-scan examination will show that the posterior cortex of the vertebral body

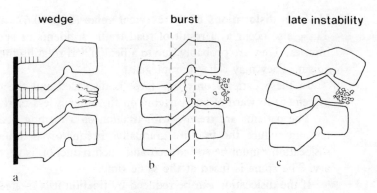

wedge   burst   late instability

Fig. 10.7. Fractures of the cervical spine

has been disrupted. Fragments of bone can be extruded backwards causing a neurological lesion (Fig. 10.7b), either a complete tetraplegia or an incomplete lesion. Furthermore because of the comminution the spine is liable to become unstable collapsing anteriorly as it heals (Fig. 10.7c).

These patients should therefore be treated by traction on a turning bed initially. If there is still significant residual neurological deficit it is reasonable to decompress these lesions from the front and incorporate a bone graft anteriorly.

If the patient is completely tetraplegic the operation will probably only increase stability of the neck and make nursing easier.

Patients without neurological deficit can be treated conservatively with traction for some weeks. Then they should be immobilised in a minerva plaster or cervical brace until the neck is stable.

However, these fractures may heal with so much collapse that later instability may occur and they then require spinal fusion.

★★★ **Hyperextension injuries** (Fig. 10.8)
A hyperextension force occurs frequently in road traffic accidents. This involves damage to the muscles anterior to the cervical spine and also to the anterior ligament. The patient complains of neck pain and exhibits tenderness over the anterior aspect of the neck. The X-ray is normal. Neurological com-

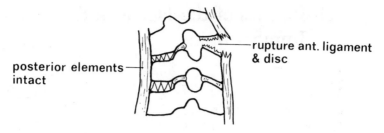

Fig. 10.8. Hyperextension injury (whiplash)

plications do not occur in a previously normal spine but may be seen in patients with cervical spondylosis.

These lesions will heal with rest and immobilisation in a collar for some weeks. Mobilising exercises may be indicated after this.

A more severe injury will involve the intervertebral disc and possibly cause a fracture of the pedicle and lamina. A kissing fracture may be found of adjacent cervical spines.

These more severe injuries require more prolonged immobilisation in a stiff collar. The fractures always heal and the disc spaces often fuse spontaneously.

Late instability is rarely a problem with these injuries if treated by immobilisation.

** **Fractures of the cervical spines**
These can occur as a result of local muscle violence. They have been called 'clay shovellers' fractures and are stable. Treatment is symptomatic using a soft collar.

11 Injuries of the Dorsal and Lumbar Spine

Compression fractures
Fractures of transverse processes
Flexion-rotation injuries
Flexion injuries (seat-belt fractures)
Pathological fractures

Most fractures of the dorsal and lumbar spine are neither severe nor complicated. They are usually stable. However, the patients are often excessively concerned and far too aware of the danger of paraplegia.

INSTABILITY

Fractures of the dorsal and lumbar spine can be unstable in a manner similar to that described for cervical spine injuries. They can be classified as either stable or unstable injuries.

Stable fractures include wedge compression fractures and fractures of the transverse processes. These require only simple treatment.

Unstable lesions include fracture dislocations of the spine (simple dislocations are almost unknown in the dorsal and lumbar region). These require careful management. Unstable injuries of the dorsal spine are usually accompanied by paraplegia.

NEUROLOGICAL COMPLICATIONS

The spinal cord ends at the first lumbar vertebra in adults (Fig. 11.1). The dura continues to the second sacral vertebra. The verterbal canal in the lumbar region contains only cauda equina nerve roots.

A displaced fracture or dislocation of the lumbar spine may well not be associated with any neurological deficit.

The dorsal vertebral canal is narrow. Any displaced fracture-

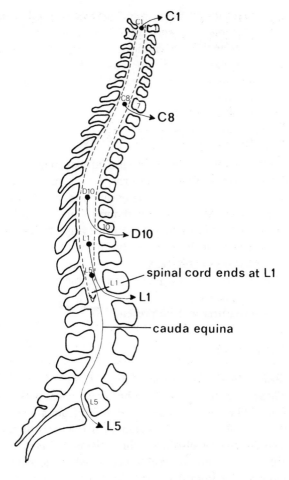

Fig. 11.1. Relationship of the spinal cord to the vertebrae

dislocation of the dorsal spine is likely to produce irreversible paraplegia.

A complete paraplegia is irreversible. If the lesion is incomplete, recovery can occur. A patient with a spinal injury must be very carefully examined to exclude any sparing of neurological function — particularly of the distal segments of the cord. A patient with a complete paraplegia is treated as such. Management of the damaged spine takes second place.

Operative decompression will not relieve a complete para-

115

plegia. In fact it is contra-indicated as it may make the spine more unstable and more difficult to manage.

Operation may be indicated to improve stability by open reduction, fixation and spinal fusion. Operation is also indicated if an incomplete neurological lesion shows signs of becoming more severe.

VISCERAL COMPLICATIONS

Fractures of the lower dorsal and lumbar spine can be associated with retroperitoneal haemorrhage or actual damage to abdominal viscera. The retroperitoneal haemorrhage will show itself as an ileus with a distended abdomen and absent bowel sounds. A ruptured viscus will have similar symptoms and the diagnosis is difficult to make in severely injured patients.

Fractures of the transverse processes of the first and second lumbar vertebrae are particularly liable to be associated with kidney damage.

Haematuria will be present.

Compression fractures

★★ *Wedge compression fractures* (Fig. 11.2a)

These occur commonly in the dorsal spine and upper lumbar spine. They occur usually after a fall from a height landing on the heels (they are associated with fractures of the os calcis). These fractures also occur in patients involved in road traffic accidents. They are easily overlooked if the patient has other more severe injuries.

The cancellous bone of the vertebral body becomes compressed within itself. The posterior ligament complex, the facet joints and the intervertebral disc are undamaged. There is no tendency for more displacement to occur and the fracture is stable.

On examination the patient is tender at the level of the fracture. There may be a slight kyphus. There are never any neurological signs. The patient may have a transient ileus.

The patient should be admitted to hospital for bed rest and for observation. After one or two weeks the acute symptoms will have subsided and active exercises are prescribed. The patient should be able to return to work in a few weeks. However, actual return to work is variable and appears to bear no relation to the severity of crushing as seen on X-ray.

*** *Bursting compression fractures* (Fig. 11.2b)
These fractures also occur after falls from a height or after road traffic accidents.

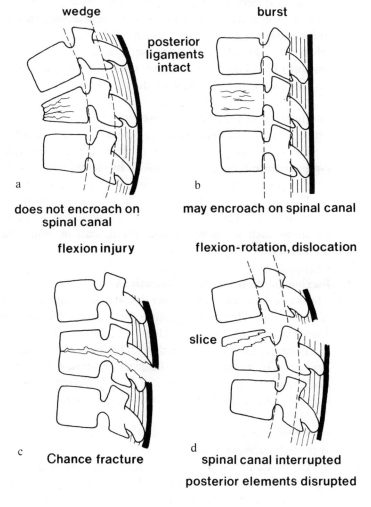

Fig. 11.2. Fractures of the dorsal or lumbar spine

The vertebral body is burst rather than compressed within itself. A CAT-scan examination will show that the posterior cortex of the vertebral body has been disrupted. The contents of the vertebral body are extruded and may go backwards into the vertebral canal and impinge on the spinal cord or nerve roots. These fractures can cause total or incomplete paraplegia. Treatment depends on the severity of the neurological deficit. If there is no neurological deficit, the patient can be treated with a short period of bed rest and then active exercises when the fracture is stable. Patients with these fractures should be followed-up carefully in the months after fracture as the vertebra has a tendency to collapse as it heals. An unacceptable amount of kyphosis can result. A spinal fusion operation may be indicated to try and prevent this.

** **Fractures of transverse processes**
These occur commonly. They may be due to direct violence.

These fractures are stable and the patient can be treated symptomatically with rest followed by active exercises. The time off work should only be a few weeks.

The fractures can be multiple and associated with other severe injuries. They may be associated with abdominal complications such as retroperitoneal haematoma or contusion of the kidney.

*** **Flexion-rotation fracture dislocations**
These injuries occur in the lower dorsal and dorsilumbar region of the spine. They result from a flexion and rotation force. They result from mining accidents and road traffic accidents.

These fractures are unstable. The posterior complex of ligaments is disrupted and the facet joints are fractured or dislocated. There is an associated 'slice' fracture through the superior part of the vertebral body immediately inferior (Fig. 11.2d).

These lesions are usually associated with a complete irreversible paraplegia.

On examination the patient may have paralysis of both lower limbs and sensory loss below the level of the lesion. There may be a band of hyperaesthesia at the level of the lesion. The back shows a localised area of bruising and swelling

between the spines at the level of the fracture. There will also
be a palpable gap opened up between the spines.

If there are no significant neurological complications the
patient is treated recumbent on a turning bed for ten weeks
and then gradually mobilised wearing a plaster jacket. In due
course the fracture dislocation will fuse spontaneously.

If the fracture dislocation is considerably displaced (especially
if there is significant lateral displacement) open reduction and
fixation with rods and spinal fusion can be performed.

*** **Fracture dislocation due to flexion mechanism (seat-belt
fractures)**

These occur in car passengers after road traffic accidents;
particularly if they wear only lap seat belts. They are usually
seen in the lumbar region. Such fractures are unstable. Two
types are described:

1 A disruption of the posterior ligament complex associated
with a crush fracture of the superior portion of the vertebra
below. X-ray will show separation of the spines and separation
of the facet joints.

2 A transverse fracture passing through the spine, pedicles
and body permitting separation of the posterior elements. This
lesion is easily seen on X-rays as a Chance fracture (Fig. 11.2c).

There may be neurological lesions associated with these
fractures. Fortunately as they occur in the lumbar region,
only nerve roots are involved and recovery is likely. These
fractures are also associated with severe abdominal lesions
which may be difficult to diagnose.

On examination of the spine a bruised swollen area can be
palpated at the level of the lesion. There may be a palpable gap
between the spines. These patients should be immobilised
lying flat on a turning bed for about ten weeks. Following this
they can be gradually mobilized wearing a plaster jacket.

If the lesion does not stabilise spontaneously operation for
spinal fusion is indicated.

Pathological fractures (Fig. 11.3)

These present commonly in the spine. The usual lesion is a
wedge compression fracture in the lower dorsal region. The

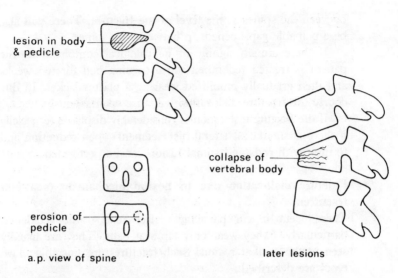

lesion in body & pedicle

collapse of vertebral body

erosion of pedicle

a.p. view of spine

later lesions

Fig. 11.3. Secondary deposits in the spine

patient complains of a sudden onset of incapacitating back pain. There is usually no history of significant trauma.

The common cause in elderly women is osteoporosis. This can only be diagnosed after excluding other lesions such as secondary metastases and myelomatosis.

The patient is admitted to hospital and treated symptomatically with bed rest. Blood investigations should include full blood count, sedimentation rate, alkaline phosphatase and plasma proteins.

If the lesion is due to secondary metastases, radiotherapy or treatment with cytotoxic drugs can be prescribed. If it is due to myelomatosis specific treatment can be organised.

Patients with osteoporosis should be mobilised as soon as possible. Treatment with Vitamin D and calcium supplements may be helpful. A surgical corset may alleviate the feeling of back weakness.

12 Paraplegia and Tetraplegia

The majority of these cases result from trauma. Other conditions such as multiple sclerosis, ascending myelitis, tumours and infections can produce a more gradual progressive lesion.

Fractures of the dorsal spine with significant displacement almost inevitably produce a complete paraplegia, as the vertebral canal is so narrow in this region. These patients have a complete paralysis of their lower limbs. Initially this paralysis is flaccid (a state of 'spinal shock') but over a period of weeks it converts to a spastic paralysis. Reflex activity returns to the intact segments of the spinal cord distal to the lesion. There is complete sensory loss. All modalities are affected, touch, pain and position sense. In a complete lesion there will be no recovery for these modalities. There is initially complete loss of bladder and bowel function. After a few weeks, reflex activity also returns to bladder and bowel function — an automatic bladder results.

Fractures of the lumbar spine will only cause neurological lesions if they are grossly displaced. These lesions are incomplete and will affect the nerve roots of the cauda equina (the spinal cord ends at the level of the first lumbar vertebra in adults) (Fig. 11.1). The nerve supply to the bladder and bowel is involved so distally that reflex activity will not return and function depends on intrinsic activity — an autonomous bladder results.

Fractures and dislocation of the cervical spine may produce a tetraplegia, affecting upper limbs as well as lower limbs. In addition, the patients have a disturbance of function of the autonomic nervous system — they develop paralytic ileus or a profound hypotension. The severity of the lesion of the upper limbs depends on the level of the injury to the cervical spine. A patient with an injury at C3/4 level may well have no function in the upper limbs or chest and may require assisted respiration in order to survive. The commonest lesion is at C5/6 level. At this level the C6 nerve root may or may not be functional and the residual capacity varies accordingly.

A patient who is completely paraplegic on admission will probably show no neurological recovery. Unfortunately at present, no form of treatment will alter this. A patient with an incomplete lesion may improve. A careful neurological examination should be made to detect any signs of an incomplete lesion such as toe movement or sparing of sacral sensation. Operative decompression of the spinal cord is only indicated if an incomplete lesion appears to be getting worse.

INITIAL MANAGEMENT

It is essential not to inflict further damage on moving these patients. They should be carried in 'one straight piece' with the spine extended at the fracture. Three persons are required to lift and one more is necessary to supervise. Four people are required to lift a tetraplegic patient — the supervisor holding the head and keeping the neck in extension.

These patients ideally should travel flat on their backs with pressure areas supported by pillows and the fracture maintained in extension. Unfortunately they often have other injuries and in order to maintain a good airway, they have to be put in a modified coma position with spine straight and supported with pillows. The care of the skin must start from injury. Pressure sores develop rapidly as the patient is paralysed and has no pain or touch sensation. The position should be changed every two hours and pressure points protected.

The fractures are usually managed conservatively. Those of the dorsal and lumbar spine can be reduced by hyper-extension over pillows and maintained adequately. Fractures and dislocations of the cervical spine can be reduced by skull traction and the reduction so maintained. Skull traction is via calipers inserted into the outer table of the skull. These patients can be treated on a turning bed. Only patients with gross malalignment require open reduction and internal fixation.

The bladder requires care to prevent over distension of the paralysed detrusor muscle. Catheterisation must be performed under very strict aseptic conditions to prevent infection. It will be some weeks before a reflex bladder can empty itself.

DEFINITIVE MANAGEMENT

Definitive management of paraplegic patients requires a centre with special facilities and special staff. These people require special nursing and special rehabilitation. The overall prognosis has improved dramatically since the need for special facilities has been appreciated. Meticulous care of the skin is essential to prevent sores. These patients in the early stages require turning every two hours — this demands either a three man team or a special turning bed. Pressure sores once present are very difficult to eradicate. Furthermore they will initiate reflex spasms and cause postural problems and eventually contractures. A patient in a wheelchair must be taught to change his position every hour to prevent pressure sores. Particular care must be taken in fitting footwear and any special appliances.

The bladder must be retrained. After injury the detrusor muscle is completely paralysed — in due course reflex contractions will return but there will be no central control. The patient can learn to initiate the contraction in various ways. Ideally there should be as low a residual urine as possible. Bladder training involves:

1 Regular catheterisation (or use of a special indwelling catheter) until a reflex bladder is established.
2 Avoidance of infection in the urinary tract.
3 Rapid treatment of infection when it occurs.
4 Establishing a reflex bladder with as low a residual urine as possible.
5 Control of incontinence.

Unfortunately most patients have some residual bladder and bowel problems. These are very severe in those with a persistently paralysed or autonomous bladder (as seen in those with cauda equina lesions).

These patients initially have a complete paralysis of bowel function. They require persistent treatment with enemas and manual evacuation until reflex activity returns. When this happens it is possible for the patient to learn how to stimulate reflex defaecation.

Intensive physiotherapy is necessary for these patients:

1 To prevent contractures and deformities:
   by daily passive movement of all joints;

by careful positioning of paralysed limbs;
by use of splints.

2 Development of upper limb and trunk muscles as soon as the initial fracture has stabilised. This has to be done gradually to avoid problems of postural hypotension. These muscles are developed in order to:
permit sitting;
allow transfer from bed, etc., to wheelchair;
allow standing in braces to help kidney and bowel function.

3 Tetraplegic patients may have problems with respiratory function requiring treatment.

Rehabilitation means adaptation:
of the patient to his disability;
of the patient's residual capacities to new functions;
of the patient's environment to accommodate him.

His waking hours will be spent predominantly in a wheelchair which can be adapted to his needs. His house and garden must be adapted to accommodate him in a wheelchair. If his employer will not accept him, the patient is trained in skills that will be accepted. Certain recreations are denied him, he is taught new ones.

13 Fractures of the Pelvis

AP compression ⎫
lat   "   ⎬ mechanism of fracture
vertical shear ⎭

** Fractures which do not disrupt the pelvic ring:
   muscle avulsion fractures
   isolated fractures of the ilium
   fractures of the ischium and/or pubic ramus on one side
      only
   isolated fractures of the sacrum
   fractures of the coccyx
*** Fractures which disrupt the pelvic ring:
   fractures of the ischium and pubic ramus on each side
   compression fractures of the pelvis
   vertical fractures of the pelvis
Fractures of the acetabulum (see Fig. 14.2)

The pelvis is in the shape of a ring. It is made up of the sacrum joined to the innominate bones at the sacroiliac joints. The pubic bones are joined together by the pubic symphysis.

Force is transmitted from the acetabulum to the sacroiliac joint by a strong column of bone in the ilium. The ischio-pubic ramus in front of the pelvis acts as an anterior tie.

It takes considerable force to disrupt the ring of the pelvis — such as results from compression injuries or falls from a height. Less severe fractures occur as a result of direct violence, leverage from the lower limb, or muscle avulsion injuries.

Fractures which disrupt the ring are liable to be complicated by excessive blood loss, damage to the urethra or other viscera, and damage to the sacroiliac joint.

Clinically, fractures of the pelvis can be difficult to diagnose. Some patients have obvious fractures with bruising and swelling around the perineum and lower abdomen. They may have tenderness over the fracture, and springing of the iliac crest may cause pain and produce crepitus. In patients with multiple injuries the only sign may be an unexplained hypovolaemic shock with blood loss. Some patients have only vague pain and an inability to stand or walk.

An X-ray of the pelvis should be taken of all patients with

multiple injuries and all patients with a serious fractures of the femur or tibia. Some fractures may be difficult to determine on A-P views, and oblique X-rays should be taken.

COMPLICATIONS

Hypovolaemic shock
The pelvis is formed of very vascular cancellous bone and is lined by numerous thin walled veins and small arteries. Excessive bleeding can result from a fracture of the pelvis that disrupts the ring. Some patients require 30−40 units of blood to replace the loss and some literally bleed to death. In due course bleeding from small vessels will cease.

Large vessels are only occasionally damaged. Exploration of these seriously ill patients is only indicated if there is evidence of large artery damage or an associated ruptured viscus.

Ruptured urethra
The posterior urethra is frequently damaged just proximal to the urogenital diaphragm. This lesion occurs in association with fracture of the pubis or separation of the pubic symphysis.

The patient may present with bleeding at the urethral meatus. They also have retention of urine. This lesion should be suspected in all patients with fractures of the pubis. A retrograde-urethrogram is probably the most useful radiological investigation.

If diagnosed a ruptured urethra should be splinted with an indwelling catheter and a suprapubic cystostomy set up to divert the urine.

Injuries to other viscera
Ruptures of the rectum and the bladder are also described. Occasionally injuries to the sigmoid colon accompany fractures of the blade of the ilium. A fractured pelvis often is only a part of a series of multiple injuries. Intraperitoneal injuries frequently coexist and should be diagnosed. Peritoneal aspiration or lavage is helpful — frequently a laparotomy is necessary to diagnose and then treat the lesion.

Neurological lesions
These occur occasionally in association with fractures involving the sacrum. Usually the lowermost nerve roots are involved.

Back pain
Patients frequently have persistent low back pain after recovering from fractures of the pelvis. This is more common after lesions involving the sacroiliac joint.

Usually this pain resolved with time. Occasionally symptoms are so severe and so persistent that a bony fusion of the sacroiliac joint is performed.

Impotence
Male patients with fractures of the pelvis may complain of impotence.

Malunion
Accurate reduction of pelvic fractures is not necessary. Union occurs adequately enough for reasonable function. It is however widely considered that a previously fractured pelvis is likely to cause damage during child birth. Elective Caesarian section is frequently performed.

Fractures which do not disrupt the pelvic ring

** *Muscle avulsion fractures*
These usually occur as a result of athletic injuries in adolescence. The patient complains of localised pain after a sudden effort. There is localised tenderness at the fracture site and X-ray will show an avulsion fracture. The common sites for avulsion fractures of the pelvis are (Fig. 13.1c):
> anterior superior iliac spine — sartorius, tensorfascia lata;
> anterior inferior iliac spine — rectus femoris;
> ischial tuberosity — hamstrings.

Treatment is rest and the symptoms will gradually resolve.

** *Isolated fractures of the ilium* (Fig. 13.1a)
These occur as the result of direct violence. The patient has an area of bruising and swelling over the iliac crest. Treatment is

127

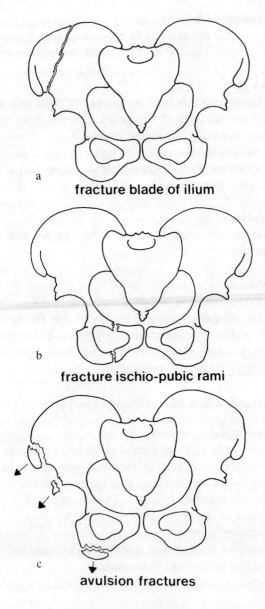

Fig. 13.1.   Fractures of the pelvis without disruption of ring

Fractures of the Pelvis

rest and the patient should be kept in hospital for few days for observation to exclude any intraperitoneal injury.

** *Fractures of the ischium and/or pubic ramus one side only* (Fig. 13.1b)
These occur frequently as the only fracture. There may be no obvious physical signs. The patient complains of pain in the pelvis and is not able to bear weight or walk.

Treatment is bed rest for two weeks followed by mobilisation with crutches. Convalescence lasts only a few weeks.

If these fractures are at all displaced it is likely that there is some associated lesion around the sacroiliac joint. The prognosis for persisting low back pain should be guarded.

*** *Isolated fractures of the sacrum*
These are seen only occasionally. Isolated fractures are undisplaced and the patient complains of back pain.

Treatment is bed rest for two weeks followed by mobilizing exercises.

Displaced fractures of the sacrum occur in conjunction with other fractures of the pelvis. These fractures are very rarely associated with damage to the sacral nerve roots.

*** *Fractures of the coccyx*
These occur after falls in the sitting position. Even though the coccyx is trivial the patient may suffer severe low back pain which is resistant to treatment.

Treatment is bed rest. If the symptoms are very persistent a coccygectomy may afford some relief.

*** **Fractures with disruption of the pelvic ring**

*** *Fractures of ischium and pubic rami on each side* (Fig. 13.2a)
These result in a floating segment anteriorly. Injuries to the posterior urethra are frequently associated with this lesion. These fractures usually result from compression forces. The fracture may only be a part of a complex of injuries in a severely ill patient.

Treatment of hypovolaemic shock and the damaged urethra take priority. The fractures will heal in reasonable position

129

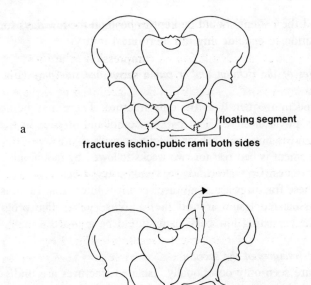

a

floating segment

fractures ischio-pubic rami both sides

b

diastasis of symphysis & fracture sacroiliac region

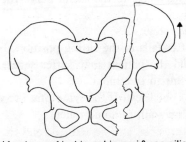

c

displaced fractures of ischio-pubic rami & sacroiliac region

Fig. 13.2. Fractures of the pelvis and disruption of ring

with rest in bed. As the ring is disrupted these patients require rest for about six weeks before mobilising with crutches.

An external fixateur can be used to stabilise these fractures. The pins are inserted into the iliac crests on each side of the pelvis. The bar lies anterior to the lower abdomen. The patients are much more comfortable and can be mobilised sooner.

*** *Fractures with separation of the pubic symphysis and separation at or near the sacroiliac joint* (Fig. 13.2b)

These fractures also result from a compression injury and the ring is opened up. There is always a separation at or near the pubic symphysis. The sacroiliac joint is subluxed or there is a fracture through the adjacent bone.

There is usually severe hypovolaemic shock due to blood loss. The posterior urethra is often damaged and other injuries are common.

The patient will require treatment for blood loss and management of the associated injuries.

The fractured segment can usually be controlled adequately with skeletal traction of the Hamilton Russell type. Reasonable alignment of the fractures usually result (see Fig. 2.6).

These fractures can also be well reduced and fixed using an external fixateur.

*** *Displaced fractures of the ischio-pubic rami associated with displacement at or near the sacroiliac joint* (Fig. 13.2c)

These usually occur as a result of falls from a height. The damaged segment is vertically displaced — the lower limb on the affected side has apparent (but not true) shortening. These patients are also severely shocked and may have other severe injuries.

The pelvis can be brought into alignment by skeletal traction on the affected side. Hamilton Russell type traction is usually the most appropriate.

The patient will require rest in bed for at least eight weeks before mobilising with crutches.

These fractures can also be reduced and the position maintained using an external fixateur.

14 Injuries of the Hip Joint

Dislocations of the hip
Fractures of the acetabulum

** **Posterior dislocation of the hip**
This is a serious injury. It frequently occurs after road traffic accidents. If the patient is seated, force is transmitted via the knee to the femur and thence to the hip joint dislocating it posteriorly (Fig. 2.1).

Injuries to the knee or the femur on the same side are common. The knee must be carefully examined and X-rayed to exclude them. When the patient is anaesthetised to reduce the hip, the opportunity should be taken to stress the knee to exclude posterior cruciate ligament injury.

When the hip is dislocated posteriorly the lower limb takes up a characteristic position. It is internally rotated, adducted and flexed (Fig. 14.1a). When a hip dislocation is associated with fractures of the femur or the tibia on the same side this position is not obvious. It is best to X-ray the pelvis of all

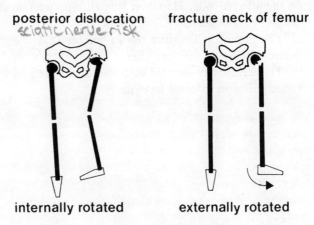

posterior dislocation   fracture neck of femur
sciatic nerve risk

internally rotated   externally rotated

Fig. 14.1.   Dislocation of the femur neck

132

patients with a serious fracture of the femur or the tibia to exclude hip dislocation or a fracture of the pelvis.

A dislocated hip may be associated with a fracture of the posterior rim of the acetabulum. This may make the reduction unstable. It is reasonable to operate on such fracture dislocations to reduce the hip and fix acetabular fragments with a screw. Other fracture fragments can occur and cause the femoral head to be incompletely reduced. Such fragments can arise from the femoral head as well as from the acetabulum. A CAT-scan examination is useful to detect such fragments.

Complications

1 Sciatic nerve palsy. The sciatic nerve is a close posterior relation of the hip joint and may be damaged as it dislocates.

The patient usually has a lesion of the tibial portion. There is loss of sensation in the sole of the foot and loss of plantar flexion movement. The lesion may involve the whole nerve in which case there will be no active movement below the knee.

The nerve usually recovers after reduction of the dislocation, although complete recovery may take some months.

2 Irreducible dislocation. It may not be possible to reduce the dislocation by manipulation and open reduction is often necessary. This may be due to:

button-holing of posterior capsule by the head of the femur
the presence of bone fragments in the hip joint

3 Recurrence of dislocation. This may occur after a fracture dislocation. It has also been described in otherwise uncomplicated dislocations.

4 Avascular necrosis. The blood supply of the head of the femur may be damaged on dislocation of the hip. Avascular necrosis of the head may supervene.

This may not cause symptoms for two or three years after dislocation. X-rays then will show sclerosis of the head and a portion may be collapsed. The patient complains of pain in the hip which is often intolerable. Operative treatment is usually necessary.

Treatment

A dislocated hip requires reduction as soon as possible. This is done under general anaesthesia in an operating theatre as manipulative reduction frequently fails. X-ray control is necessary and a good A-P and lateral view must be taken.

It is easy to reduce the dislocation partially and care must be taken in interpreting the films.

Following reduction the hip is best immobilised with Hamilton Russell type traction for three weeks before allowing the patient to mobilise with crutches (Fig. 2.6).

*** **Anterior dislocation of the hip**
Nowadays this lesion is uncommon. The head of the femur dislocates forwards. The leg appears externally rotated — a position similar to a fracture of the neck of the femur (Fig. 14.1b).

*** **Fracture dislocation of the hip**
A fracture of the posterior lip of the acetabulum is frequently associated with a posterior dislocation. If the fragment is large it should be replaced at operation and fixed with a screw.

Fractures of the femoral head or acetabulum may become displaced into the acetabulum and hinder reduction.

Sometimes after the reduction they act as loose bodies and cause rapid onset of degenerative changes in the hip. These loose fragments should be removed by operation.

Fractures of the acetabulum
These fractures can occur from a force transmitted to the acetabulum via the greater trochanter such as occurs when a pedestrian is knocked down by a car. They may also occur from a force transmitted up the leg to the shaft of the femur — as in falls from a height (Fig. 14.2a).

The head of the femur impacts on to the acetabulum and fragments it. Degenerative changes occur frequently as late complications after these fractures.

** *Undisplaced fractures of the acetabulum* occur fairly frequently. The patient complains of pain and stiffness in the hip. There are often other injuries to the limb on the same side or the patient may have generalised severe injuries.

The fracture is often difficult to demonstrate on A-P X-ray of the hip and oblique views may be necessary. A CAT-

134

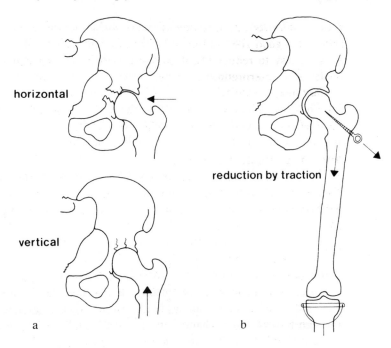

horizontal

vertical

reduction by traction

a   b

Fig. 14.2.   Mechanisms of acetabular fracture

scan examination adds a third dimension and is often invaluable in confirming the diagnosis and elucidating the severity of the fracture.

These patients are best treated in bed, the affected limb immobilised with skin traction for three weeks. After this the patients can be mobilised non-weight bearing for another three weeks.

Degenerative changes may occur sooner or later after these fractures and cause incapacitating symptoms.

*** *Fractures of the posterior rim of the acetabulum*
These are often associated with a dislocated hip but may occur as isolated injuries.

If the fractures are small they can be managed by bed rest and skin traction. However if the fragments are large they are best reduced by open reduction and fixation with a screw.

Chapter 14

**** *Displaced fractures of the acetabulum (central dislocations)*
These are very severe injuries to the hip joint. The injury is
more severe than represented on X-ray as the articular cartilage
is also fragmented and torn away. Degenerative changes in the
hip are almost inevitable.

These lesions can be classified by the degree of the displacement of the fragments. They can also be classified as to which
portion of the acetabulum — ilio-pubic or ilio-ischial — is
involved.

Ideally these fractures should be reduced anatomically and
fixed with plates and screws. Unfortunately these patients often
have other severe injuries which take priority. The operation is
very difficult and frequently the fractures are so comminuted
that an anatomical reduction is not possible. It has yet to be
shown that the long term results from these operations are
better than those obtained by more conservative methods.

In practice most of these fractures are treated by traction.
Two planes of traction can be used. One is by a screw fixed
through the greater trochanter and passing laterally. The other
is along the line of the limb via skeletal traction through the
tibial tuberosity (Fig. 14.2b).

The position of the fragments is improved. Traction is
continued for six weeks. The patient is then mobilised non-
weight bearing on crutches for a further six weeks.

15 Fractures of the Neck of the Femur

*** Fractures of the neck of the femur in the elderly
    subcapital fractures
    per- or inter-trochanteric fractures
    subtrochanteric fractures
*** Fractures of the neck of the femur in young people (or children)
    cervical fractures
    subtrochanteric fractures
    acute slip of upper femoral epiphysis

These fractures occur only too commonly in elderly people who suffer from osteoporosis. Osteoporosis is a condition associated with a reduction in bone mass and a decreased production of osteoid. The chemical composition of the bone is normal. X-ray will show increased radiolucency with thinning of the calcar. The femoral neck is weakened and fractures occur after minimal or non-existent trauma.

These fractures are also found in debilitated people and alcoholics, whose bones are also osteoporotic.

Pathological fractures occur at the site of secondary deposits and also occur in patients with Paget's disease.

Fractures of the neck of the femur only occasionally occur in young people. In these patients they are high energy fractures resulting from road traffic accidents or falls from a height.

All patients with fractures of the neck of femur complain of a painful hip. There is usually very little in the way of bruising and swelling. If the fracture is displaced the leg is short and lies in external rotation (Fig. 14.1b). However, if the fracture is undisplaced the leg will remain in neutral position. It must be remembered that it is possible to walk on an undisplaced fracture of the neck of the femur, although it will cause pain.

A good A-P and lateral X-ray is necessary to make the diagnosis. An undisplaced subcapital fracture of the neck of the femur is sometimes very difficult to visualise. It is quite permissible to admit an old lady with a painful hip to hospital for a few days and then repeat X-ray to exclude such a fracture. A bone scan may indicate the diagnosis of fracture.

Fractures of the neck of the femur take about three or four months to unite satisfactorily. They can be treated with traction for that length of time — a type of Hamilton Russell traction is useful.

However, old people when confined to bed for any length of time tend to develop various complications:

deep vein thrombosis and pulmonary embolism
'hypostatic pneumonia'
urinary retention and infections
bedsores
psychiatric disturbances
worsening osteoporosis

The morbidity and mortality of this condition is greatly reduced by fixing these fractures internally to permit early mobilisation. Young people are usually unwilling to rest in bed for three months and they prefer operation to fix their frac-ures.

Displaced subcapital fractures in the elderly and cervical fractures in the young are best managed by open reduction. The incidence of delayed union and avascular necrosis is reduced.

Fractures of the neck of the femur in the elderly

Subcapital fractures
These can be displaced or undisplaced. A fracture through the neck of the femur in the subcapital region is liable to damage the posterior-lateral artery. This is the main blood supply to the head of the femur.

If the blood supply of the head is disrupted the fracture may progress to non-union. Even if the fracture eventually unites the head may die and progress to avascular necrosis (Fig. 15.1).

Avascular necrosis may not become apparent clinically for months or even years. The patient complains of gradually in-creasing pain in the hip. X-ray will show the head of the femur as being more dense with an area of collapse. Symptoms may be so severe that operative treatment — often a total hip replacement — is necessary.

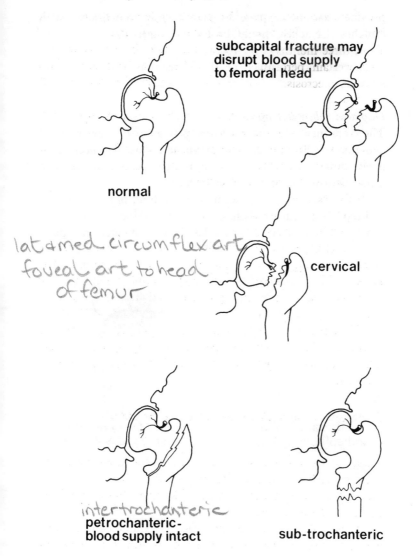

Fig. 15.1. Fractures of the femur neck

Undisplaced subcapital fractures may progress to avascular necrosis, displaced fractures often do.

*** *Undisplaced subcapital fractures*
These are best fixed in elderly people to permit early mobilisation. Threaded pins or cancellous screws may be used and will

139

provide fixation adequate to permit early mobilisation with crutches. Crutches should be retained until union occurs in about three months (Fig. 15.2a).

A certain percentage of these fractures will proceed to avascular necrosis.

*** *Displaced subcapital fractures*

These are unsatisfactory fractures to treat. If they are reduced and pinned the rate of non-unioin and avascular necrosis is greater than 50%. A more complicated fixation device than screws is usually considered necessary.

It is reasonable to excise the femoral head in these patients and replace it with a prosthesis. An Austin-Moore or Thomson prosthesis is often used — the last being cemented into place (Fig. 12.2b).

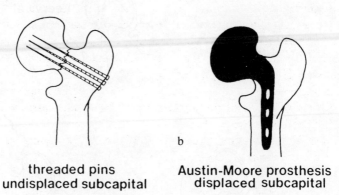

a

**threaded pins
undisplaced subcapital**

b

**Austin-Moore prosthesis
displaced subcapital**

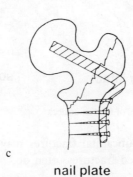

c

**nail plate
pertrochanteric**

Fig. 15.2. Fixation of fractures of the femur neck

The operation has its own complications but is a worthwhile procedure in the elderly. After a few days the patient can walk with crutches.

*** *Pertrochanteric fractures*

These fractures occur through cancellous bone and unite readily. The fracture is well distal to the blood supply of the head of the femur and avascular necrosis is not a complication (Fig. 15.1).

These fractures take three months to unite treated by traction. They are best treated by operation — a nail is inserted into the head under X-ray control and a plate secured to it and screwed on to the shaft. This fixation is adequate to permit protected weight bearing a few days after operation (Fig. 15.2c).

*** *Subtrochanteric fractures*

These are really fractures of the upper femoral shaft and occur through cortical bone (Fig. 15.1). They are less common and often produced by more severe violence such as road traffic accidents. Old people with these fractures are best treated by operation.

Fractures of the neck of the femur in young people

*** *Cervical fractures*

Such fractures occur through the middle or the base of the neck (Fig. 15.1). They are high energy fractures occurring from falls or road traffic accidents. They may only be part of a complex of serious injuries.

Non-union of these fractures and avascular necrosis occur in a high percentage of cases. The best results are obtained by open reduction and internal fixation — threaded pins are usually used (Fig. 15.2a).

*** Subtrochanteric fractures

These are also high energy fractures. There is often considerable bruising and swelling of the overlying skin. These patients often have other severe injuries.

It may be wise to treat these patients on traction for three to four weeks before operating on the fractures. This allows repair of the overlying tissues.

*** *Acute slip of upper femoral epiphysis*
This lesion occurs in adolescents and in boys more frequently than in girls. The patient develops sudden acute pain in the hip (or knee) and is unable to bear weight. On examination the hip may lie in external rotation like a fractured neck of femur. There may be a past history of hip pain suggesting a previous mild slip.

The slip occurs between the hypertrophic and calcifying zone of the epiphyseal plate. If the slip is not severe then an operation is performed to pin the head of the femur to stabilise it. A severe slip should be manipulated only if the acute episode has occurred within a few hours. There is a very real danger of damaging the blood supply to the head of the femur and causing avascular necrosis. Otherwise the patient is treated with traction until the acute symptoms subside. The position of the leg can then be corrected by osteotomy.

16 Fractures of the Shaft of the Femur

*** Fractures of the upper and middle third of the shaft of the femur
*** Fractures of the distal third of the shaft of the femur
** Fractures of the femur in children
*** Pathological fractures of the femur

In adults fractures of the shaft of the femur can represent a very severe injury. There is often considerable damage to the surrounding soft tissues and considerable associated blood loss. There are frequently other injuries.

Compound fractures of the femur are always associated with severe soft tissue and muscle damage. The overlying skin wound may be small but it requires extensive exploration and careful debridement.

*** Fractures of the upper and middle third of the femur

First aid
These are best managed by a modified Thomas splint. The ring of the splint is fitted around the groin and the patient's foot is tied firmly to the base of the splint. The leg is thus incorporated in the splint and the patient can be transported without too much discomfort. If a Thomas splint is not available, a plank can be placed between both legs and each tied to it — splinting one leg with the other.

Emergency treatment may be required for hypovolaemic shock after serious injuries.

Conservative treatment
Fractures of the shaft of femur are best treated initially by traction. This can be set up under general anaesthesia — the opportunity being taken to manipulate the fracture into alignment at the same time.

A Steinmann pin is inserted into the tibial tubercle. The leg is immobilised in a Thomas splint with sliding traction. The lower leg rests on a knee flexion attachment (Fig. 2.5).

143

Traction can be continued until the fracture unites — at least thirteen weeks. The method requires continuous and specialised care. X-rays must be taken frequently and the weights adjusted as the fragments tend to distract. The distal femur has a tendency to swing into varus after a few weeks as the adductor muscles recover their tone.

After three months the patient can be mobilised in a simple weight-relieving caliper for two or three months. Knee stiffness is a considerable problem and a rigorous exercise programme is necessary to overcome it.

Operative treatment
If it is technically possible, internal fixation of a fractured femur saves hospital time and is much more convenient for the patient. Intramedullary fixation with a Kuntscher nail is commonly used (Fig. 2.14).

The Kuntscher nail is inserted throughout the length of the femur. It has a clover leaf cross-section which permits it to be impacted in the intermedullary canal. Length is restored and the nail is resistant to bending forces. However there is little resistance to torsion apart from the interlocking of the fracture fragments themselves.

Rehabilitation
Fractures of the shaft of the femur are associated with considerable muscle damage and considerable knee stiffness which decreases as the fracture unites. The patients require a prolonged exercise programme to regain normal function.

Patients with uncomplicated fractures of the femur may be off heavy manual work for six to nine months.

*** **Fractures of the distal third of the shaft of the femur**
Displaced fractures in this region may damage the femoral artery as it passes through the opening in the adductor magnus (Fig. 16.1b).

The femur has a wide intramedullary canal in its distal third and is not really suitable for intramedullary fixation. A blade plate may be used — this however does not afford secure enough fixation to do away with external splintage (Fig. 16.1a).

blade plate fixation

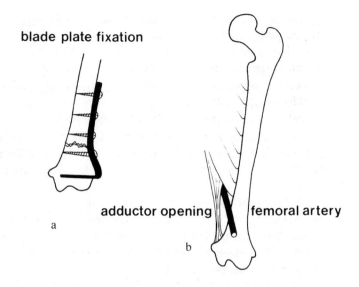

adductor opening   femoral artery

a

b

fracture distal end femur shaft

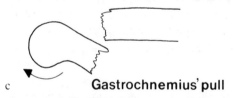

c   Gastrochnemius' pull

Fig. 16.1. Fractures of the lower third of the femur

These fractures occasionally are slow to unite and non-union does occur at this site.

Fractures of the distal third of the femur can be treated conservatively by using traction. The distal fragment becomes flexed by the gastrocnemii (Fig. 16.1c). The knee is flexed in the knee piece to accommodate for this. Traction is continued on a Thomas splint for six to eight weeks. Following this a cast-brace can be applied and the patient gradually mobilised. The cast-brace may have to be retained for some three months.

Fractures through the supracondylar region are particularly difficult to manage. The distal fragment is small and sometimes uncontrollable with traction. A badly displaced fracture may damage the popliteal artery. They are probably best fixed with a blade plate followed by a cast-brace.

** **Fractures of the femur in children**
These are common in children. They are frequently seen as an isolated injury from torsional violence and are low energy fractures which present no serious problems.

Transverse or comminuted fractures also occur which are high energy fractures and may be associated with other multiple injuries. There may be considerable blood loss requiring blood transfusion.

Fractures of the shaft of the femur unite easily in children and remodel well. It is found that, over the two years following fracture, the femur will overgrow by 1.0–1.5 cm. This overgrowth is enhanced by operating on the fracture. 1.0–1.5 cm of shortening can be accepted happily as it is eliminated by this overgrowth.

Fractured femurs in children should be treated by traction. Skin traction is usual. If skeletal traction is used the pin must *not* be inserted into the tibial tubercle. This is part of the upper tibial growth plate — damage may cause premature fusion. A disabling back knee deformity known as genu recurvatum results.

Very young children — up to three years of age — are treated by gallows traction. The strapping extensions are applied to both legs and the child is suspended via pulleys using about 2 lb weight (Fig. 2.3).

Traction should be continued until the fracture unites usually about six weeks. Alternatively a plaster spica can be applied when the fracture is stabilised after about three weeks. This usually involves a general anaesthetic but does permit the child to go home to his parents.

Older children are treated simply by fixed skin traction in a Thomas splint. A knee flexion piece is not usually necessary — knee stiffness is not such a problem in children. The anterior bow of the femur is preserved by careful padding under the fractures site to prevent it sagging.

Traction can be continued for eight to ten weeks until union has occurred. Alternatively a plaster spica can be applied after four or five weeks and retained for about two months.

The child usually requires some support for the limb after removal of the splintage. A plaster back slab is adequate.

These children will regain normal function in due course and formal physiotherapy is rarely necessary.

*** **Pathological fractures of the femur**

Secondary deposits are the commonest cause. The only way to manage these fractures is by internal fixation. The Kuntscher nail is invaluable. The fracture frequently unites after fixation — radiotherapy can be administered.

If the fracture is due to a primary tumour, a radical amputation is the best treatment.

17 Knee Joint Injuries

Management of acute knee injuries
Ligament injuries
Meniscus injuries
Injuries of the quadriceps mechanism
Fractures of the patella
Dislocations of the knee
Fractures involving the articular surface of the lower end of the femur
Fractures involving the articular surface of the upper end of the tibia

** Management of acute knee injuries

The patient presents (frequently after a sports injury) with pain and swelling of the knee. Clinical examination will reveal bruising and an effusion (a haemarthrosis). Tenderness may be elicited over the joint line or over the attachment of either the medial or lateral ligament. The pain and muscle spasm is often such that it is impossible to demonstrate ligament laxity.

In practice the management of an acute knee injury depends on the facilities available to that particular patient. An X-ray should be taken to exclude any fractures — particularly any avulsion fractures.

If the knee is not too painful and it is possible to exclude ligament laxity on clinical examination the patient can be managed with a compression bandage (possibly reinforced with a plaster slab). He should rest the limb and use crutches. In a weeks time he should be re-examined before being referred for physiotherapy.

However, if the knee is so painful that ligament laxity cannot be excluded, or if there is a large effusion, he should be examined under a general anaesthetic in an operating theatre. The haemarthrosis can be aspirated under optimum conditions. The knee can be stressed and ligament laxity noted. A stress X-ray can be taken (this is of particular value in an adolescent patient as it may be the only way of distinguishing between the

148

laxity of a ligament rupture and that of an epiphyseal fracture). If the facilities and the time are available the knee can be irrigated clear and an arthroscopy performed.

If there is a meniscus tear or a rupture of the medial ligament these lesions can be dealt with under the same anaesthetic. Management of cruciate ligament tears depends on the particular requirements of that patient. Other lesions can be adequately treated by immobilisation in a plaster cylinder for a few weeks. Following this the plaster is bivalved and the knee mobilised by exercising — the plaster slab can be retained for protection. Definitive investigation can be instituted, if necessary, after the knee has been fully mobilised.

Ligament injuries

Knee ligament injuries result from falls, athletic injuries and road traffic accidents. If they are inadequately treated there will be some laxity of the ligament and the knee will become unstable. Further secondary injuries are likely — particularly if the patient tries to continue his sporting activities. An athlete will find such a lesion particularly disabling as the knee is liable to let him down.

The knee ligaments cannot be considered in isolation. An injury to a main ligament is usually associated with damage to the joint capsule, a meniscus or another main ligament.

Ligament injuries can be classified as below (Fig. 17.1).

1 *Sprain.* The ligament is damaged but there is no detectable laxity. A mild sprain can be treated with a supporting bandage, rest and local applications. A more severe sprain is best immobilised in plaster for three weeks followed by a rigorous programme of quadriceps exercises before resuming sporting activities.

2 *Rupture in the substance of the ligament.* This is a common lesion. There is laxity of the ligament on testing clinically and the joint is unstable. The fibres of the ligament rupture individually and are teased out and stretched. At operation it is difficult to identify the torn ends and repair consists of a reefing procedure supplemented by incorporating a tendon such as that of semitendinosus.

3 *Obvious disruptions of the ligament.* This occur either at the tibial or femoral attachment. This type of injury is obviously

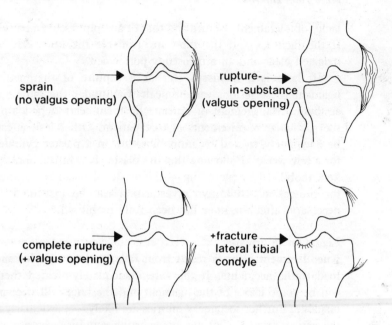

Fig. 17.1. Medial ligament injuries

best treated surgically and an accurate repair can be accomplished. Clinically, it is impossible to distinguish this lesion from a rupture in the substance of the ligament.

4 *Avulsion fractures*. These are visible on X-ray. Repair consists of reconstitution of the fracture fragments (and ligament attachments) surgically.

Lesions to be considered:
- ★★★ Medial ligament rupture
- ★★★ Lateral ligament rupture
- ★★★ Posterior cruciate ligament rupture
- ★★★ Anterior cruciate ligament rupture

★★★ *Medial ligament rupture*

A rupture of the medial ligament results from abduction violence. This can be produced by sporting injuries, road traffic accidents or falls. In older patients abduction violence tends to produce a depressed fracture of the lateral condyle — sometimes the two lesions are combined (Fig. 17.1).

An abduction injury can produce a triad of lesions known

as O'Donoghue's triad. This consists of rupture of the medial ligament, tear of the medial meniscus and rupture of the anterior cruciate (Fig. 17.2). It results in a very unstable knee if not adequately treated.

The patient with a medial ligament injury will present with a painful knee — there is often extensive bruising on the inner side. There may not be a haemarthrosis, as the joint capsule is so badly torn that it leaks away. On applying a valgus stress to the knee, laxity of the medial side can be demonstrated (Fig. 17.1).

Fit young patients develop so much muscle spasm after injury that this laxity can be difficult to demonstrate. It is best therefore to examine the knee under a general anaesthetic to exclude medial ligament rupture. It is customary to treat young patients and athletes by surgery to repair a ruptured medial ligament. More elderly people are treated by immobilisation in a plaster cylinder. They usually have surprisingly satisfactory results.

*** *Lateral ligament injuries*
Stability of the lateral side of the knee depends on the fascia lata insertion and the popliteus tendon as well as the lateral ligament proper (Fig. 17.3). Laxity of the lateral side of the knee indicates damage to these three structures. These lesions occur

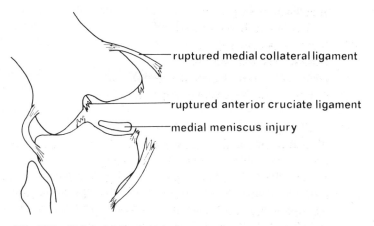

ruptured medial collateral ligament

ruptured anterior cruciate ligament

medial meniscus injury

Fig. 17.2. Triad of abduction injuries

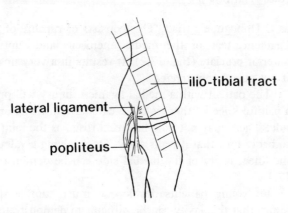

Fig. 17.3. Lateral ligament complex

from adduction violence to the knee as is seen in pedestrians knocked down by a car.

X-ray may show a fracture of the upper end of the fibula (to which the lateral ligament is attached). Sometimes the peroneal nerve is damaged and the patient has a foot-drop.

Most patients with this injury are adequately treated by immobilisation in a plaster cylinder for six weeks.

*** *Posterior cruciate ligament rupture* (Fig. 17.4)

The posterior cruciate ligament has been considered most important in controlling knee joint movements. After injury the knee may be very unstable and the patient have severe and incapacitating symptoms. However, there is considerable variation in the manner individual patients regain function after posterior cruciate injury.

Posterior cruciate injury usually follows significant injury such as a road traffic accident. It may be associated with a hip dislocation after dashboard injury. It is worthwhile stressing the knee under the same anaesthetic after reducing a dislocated hip (Fig. 2.1).

The posterior draw sign is positive. It is important to notice the contour of the knee as it tends to sag backwards if the posterior structures are ruptured — a false anterior drawer sign may be elicited. X-ray may show a small bone fragment avulsed from the posterior aspect of the upper tibia.

RUPTURE POSTERIOR CRUCIATE LIGAMENT

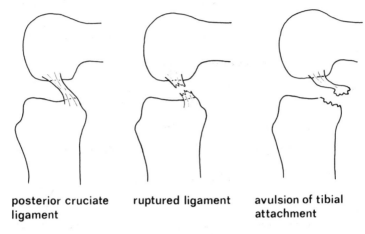

posterior cruciate   ruptured ligament   avulsion of tibial
ligament   attachment

Fig. 17.4.   Rupture of posterior cruciate ligament

These patients are probably best treated by reattaching the posterior cruciate and posterior capsule by operation. However this may not be possible as these patients often suffer other severe injuries. The lesion may be treated with plaster, and very gratifying recovery may result if the patient can regain strong quadriceps function.

*** *Anterior cruciate ligament injury* (Fig. 17.5)
This is a very common sports injury. It occurs when the patient lands awkwardly twisting his knee after jumping for the ball. He 'feels something go' in his knee. It becomes very painful and swells. Usually he has to leave the field.

On examination the knee is swollen from a haemarthrosis. There may be no other definite physical signs. Sometimes there is a block to extension movement.

The patient may have a positive drawer sign. However, this is more commonly found in patients with a chronic lesion with associated damage to the capsular ligaments of either the medial or lateral side.

In children and adolescents the injury may be associated with an avulsion of the tibial spine (the tibial attachment of the

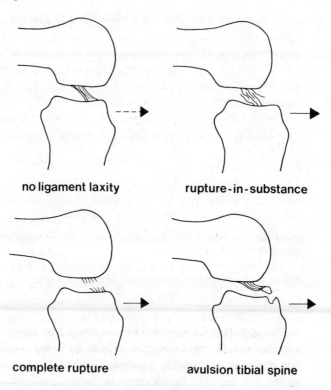

no ligament laxity   rupture-in-substance

complete rupture   avulsion tibial spine

Fig. 17.5. Rupture of anterior cruciate ligament

anterior cruciate). In these young people it is worth performing an operation and fixing the tibial spine with pins.

Usually the anterior cruciate ligament is stretched in its substance. It is probably useless to attempt an immediate suture of such a lesion. If an operation is indicated a reconstruction using part of the patella tendon or the fascia lata is done.

Theoretically, the anterior cruciate prevents the tibia sliding forward on the femur. Also, in combination with the posterior cruciate, it holds the femoral and tibial surfaces of the knee in firm apposition in all positions of the knee. If the anterior cruciate is ruptured the patient is aware of a feeling of instability when he attempts certain functions of the knee. Furthermore if he continues to play contact sports he is at risk of developing 'secondary injuries' to the menisci or the capsule.

Fortunately most functions of the knee can be accomplished without an efficient anterior cruciate ligament, provided the quadriceps and the hamstrings can be built up strongly. The patient should stop playing contact sports (including basketball and netball), however, he can run and play sports such as tennis and squash reasonably well.

If the patient must play contact sports, he can have a reconstruction operation or wear an anti-rotation brace.

*** **Meniscus lesions**

The menisci are made of fibrocartilage. They are avascular and a tear in the substance of the meniscus will probably not heal (although it has been shown that a peripheral tear can heal if it is repaired). Tears are produced by a rotation force on the flexed weight-bearing knee.

In young people, the meniscus is strong. In older people, it becomes degenerate and is more easily torn. Such tears are of a different type than those of the younger patients (Fig. 17.6).

The young patient can often give a precise history of the mechanism. It is frequently a twisting injury sustained during a sporting activity. He complains of a sudden severe pain on the side of the knee affected; it may lock and the pain is such that he has to stop playing. Over the next few hours the knee becomes swollen. The symptoms may eventually subside but are liable to recur on subsequent twisting movements of the knee.

The tear is usually longitudinal, starting in the posterior part of the meniscus and extending anteriorly. The knee is 'locked' when the central torn portion dislocates into the centre of the joint as a 'bucket-handle', this prevents full extension of the knee.

An older patient will complain of a sudden pain in the knee on kneeling or squatting. Swelling develops later. The pain and swelling persist and there may be a clicking sensation in the knee. The tear in older patients is usually horizontal and may form a tag from the posterior horn.

Meniscus tears are usually in the medial meniscus. Such medial tears usually give rise to well-localised symptoms. Tears of the lateral meniscus occur in a similar manner, however, the symptoms are often imprecise and poorly localised.

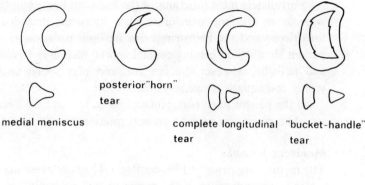

posterior "horn"
tear

medial meniscus   complete longitudinal   "bucket-handle"
                                tear   tear

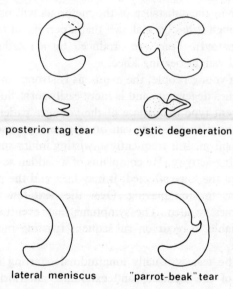

posterior tag tear   cystic degeneration

lateral meniscus   "parrot-beak" tear

Fig. 17.6. Meniscus lesions

Investigation of patients with meniscus lesions should include an X-ray to exclude other pathology. An arthroscopy is an invaluable investigation. This consists of passing an endoscope into the joint and inspecting all the compartments. With practice both menisci can be seen in their entirety.

If a meniscus is seen to be torn, the torn portion should be removed using the arthroscope. Such tears, if left, cause persistant symptoms and will cause degenerative changes to occur. It is not necessary to remove the whole meniscus, doing so affects the stability and congruity of the knee.

Injuries of the quadriceps mechanism
The quadriceps mechanism consists of:
> The four parts of the quadriceps muscle;
> The quadriceps expansion and its attachment to the patella;
> The patella and its associated retinaculum;
> The ligamentum patellae;
> The tibial tuberosity.

By direct violence
The best example of this is the dashboard injury to the occupant of a motor vehicle involved in an accident which produces a direct violence-type fracture of the patella. This tends to be a comminuted fracture which is not necessarily widely separated.

By indirect violence
Indirect violence injuries are due to a sudden contracture of the quadriceps muscle against fixed resistance. This will produce a series of injuries (Fig. 17.7):

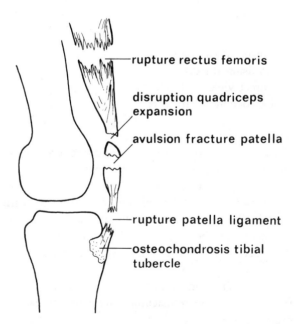

Fig. 17.7. Injuries to the quadriceps mechanism

** *Rupture of the rectus femoris* is found on occasions in young athletes after excessive exertion. They present with a swelling in the muscle. This is fairly easily repaired if the patient presents early and the lesion is diagnosed. Even if it is not repaired, function is still very good if it is managed conservatively.

*** *Rupture of the quadriceps expansion*
This occurs in elderly people. The classic cause is when the patient stumbles against the curb as he is making a stride and the quadriceps contracts and avulses itself away just at its attachment to the patella.

This is difficult to diagnose as the X-ray shows no fracture. There is considerable swelling and a palpable gap just above the patella and the patient will be unable to perform an active straight leg raise.

It is essential that the rupture is diagnosed as it requires operative repair followed by immobilisation for some weeks, in order to restore adequate function of the quadriceps and to stabilise the knee.

Fractures of the patella
> Avulsion fractures
> Direct violence fractures
> Osteochondral fractures

*** *Avulsion fractures of the patella*
These are transverse fractures and the fragments are separated by the action of the quadriceps.

These patients are best treated by an operation to fix the patella — with screws or by tension band wiring. If the fracture involves only a pole of the patella — the small fragment can be excised and the retinaculum repaired. If the fracture is very comminuted the patella is excised and the retinaculum repaired (Fig. 17.8).

A plaster cylinder is usually necessary to immobilise the fracture (and the retinaculum) for some weeks before active exercises are started.

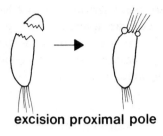

excision proximal pole

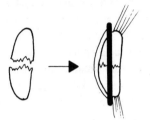

repair & tension band wire

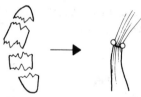

patellectomy & repair quadriceps mechanism

Fig. 17.8.   Repair of patella fractures

Direct violence fractures

Direct violence fractures of the patella are seen frequently
after road traffic accidents or after falls on the knee. There
is usually some damage to the articular surface of the knee
even in undisplaced fractures.

The patient presents with a painful knee and a haemarthrosis. The patella exhibits tenderness at the fracture site.
The fracture may be complicated later by knee stiffness and
in due course by degenerative changes in the patello-femoral
compartment of the knee.

159

** *Undisplaced fractures* should have any haemarthrosis aspirated and a plaster cylinder applied. This should be retained for six weeks. At the end of this time the plaster is bivalved and physiotherapy started — the patient retaining the back slab for comfort and protection.

** *Comminuted fractures* of the patella usually have extensive damage to the articular surface. The incidence of knee stiffness and of degenerative changes in the patello-femoral joint is high. The operation of patellectomy is usually performed for these patients.

*** *Osteochondral fractures of the patella*
These can occur as isolated injuries after direct violence or in association with a dislocated patella and may be difficult to see on X-ray.

The patient has a painful knee with a haemarthrosis. If fat globules are found in the blood-stained aspirate there may well be an osteochondral fracture. These fragments tend to persist as loose bodies and cause knee locking. They should be removed using an arthroscope if possible; a full arthrotomy may be necessary.

Dislocations of the knee

** *Dislocations of the patella* (Fig. 17.9)
The patella dislocates laterally. The dislocation can result from a twisting force after a fall, often caused by sports injuries.

In some patients it occurs easily and they are said to be subject to recurrent dislocation of the patella. Recurrent dislocation is a common sequel to a dislocation of the patella.

Some patients habitually dislocate the patella each time they flex their knees. A rare condition of congenital dislocation of the patella is described.

An osteochondral fracture may be found in association with a dislocated patella. The fragment comes from either the margin of the patella or the femoral condyle. It acts as a loose body in the knee joint and has to be removed.

The patient with a dislocation of the patella has a painful knee after a rotation injury. It may be swollen and the knee is held flexed. The patella is sometimes difficult to palpate and it is often difficult to tell if it is dislocated.

patella in groove

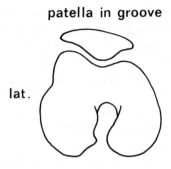

lat.

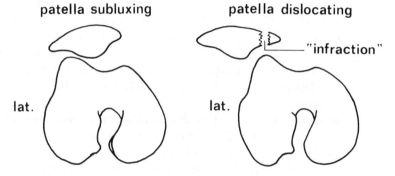

patella subluxing

lat.

patella dislocating

"infraction"

lat.

Fig. 17.9.   Dislocating patella

On extending the knee gently the patella will often reduce itself with a clunk. If the patella has been dislocated for any length of time a general anaesthetic is necessary. After reduction a plaster cylinder should be applied and retained for three weeks to stabilise the patella. Even so symptoms of recurrent dislocation or subluxation are common sequelae.

*** *Total dislocations of the knee*
Dislocation of the knee is a severe injury. Fortunately it is uncommon and usually only arises after road traffic accidents or severe violence. The politeal artery is frequently torn and there may be injury to the peroneal nerve.

Knee dislocations should be reduced as soon as possible under general anaesthetic. It is reasonable to perform an arteriogram to exclude arterial damage immediately following reduction of the dislocation. An arterial injury can be repaired at once.

After reduction of the dislocation the knee is immobilised in a plaster cylinder for six weeks and then mobilised. Surprisingly good function usually results.

Fractures involving the articular surface of the lower end of the femur

★★★ T-shaped condylar fractures
★★★ Oblique fractures of one condyle
★★★ Osteochondral or chondral fractures
★★★ Fractures through the lower femoral epiphysis

T-shaped fractures usually result from direct violence to the knee (Fig. 17.10) — sometimes from a dashboard injury in a car accident. The patella and the hip on the same side may also be damaged. There is a gross bruising and a haemarthrosis around the knee. Frequently the patient has other severe injuries. Often the lesion is compound. The knee joint should be aspirated.

★★ If the fracture is *minimally displaced* the leg can be treated with a plaster back slab and skeletal traction. When the acute symptoms have subsided, active non weight bearing exercises are instituted. After about four weeks a cast brace is applied and weight bearing commenced.

★★ If the fracture is *displaced*, open reduction and fixation with screws or a bolt should be performed in an attempt to obtain an anatomical reduction. The leg can be put in skeletal traction and treated with early movements as for an undisplaced fracture.

The main delayed complication of this fracture is knee stiffness.

The commonest late complication is the onset of degenerative changes in the knee joint.

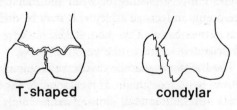

T-shaped   **condylar**

Fig. 17.10. Fractures of the articular surface of the femur

*** *Oblique fractures* may occur through either the lateral or the medial condyle (Fig. 17.10). They are seen in young athletes or motorcyclists after shearing violence. These fractures are usually displaced.

In order to restore any sort of knee function displaced condyle fractures require open reduction and fixation with bolts or screws. A pin for traction should be inserted through the upper tibia after the operation and a plaster back slab applied. After a week active movements are started non-weight-bearing and the patient treated as for a T-shaped fracture. Even though an anatomical reduction is achieved with the help of X-rays, there is always some comminution of the articular cartilage at the fracture site. There is a very real chance of these knees developing degenerative changes in later life.

Osteochondral fractures also occur as a result of sheer stress. The patients are usually young athletes or motorcyclists.

The knee becomes painful and swollen with a haemarthrosis. X-ray may not show the lesion as it is formed predominantly of cartilage. If the knee is aspirated, fat globules may be seen in the blood-stained fluid. These are diagnostic of an intra-articular fracture.

Such fractures are best treated by arthroscopy or an arthrotomy and the loose fragments removed. If they are left they will cause persistent locking.

*** *Fractures of the lower femoral epiphysis in children*
These are not uncommon and may be difficult to see on X-ray. All types of epiphyseal injury are seen. The lower femoral growth plate is the main centre for growth in the lower limb. If a complete growth arrest occurs in a young child a very severe degree of shortening will result. If an incomplete arrest occurs a severe deformity will result.

*** A type 1 injury passing between the metaphysis and growth plate occurs in teenage athletes. It may be difficult to detect on X-ray. Stress X-ray of the knee (taken under general anaesthesia) will help demonstrate it (Fig. 17.11).

The fracture should be reduced and immobilised in a plaster cylinder. Union occurs in a few weeks. In the adolescent loss of growth will be minimal — in a young child there may well be significant shortening.

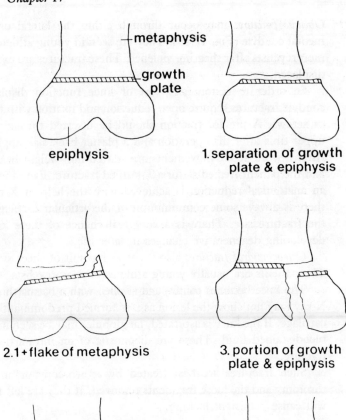

1. separation of growth plate & epiphysis

2. 1 + flake of metaphysis

3. portion of growth plate & epiphysis

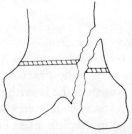

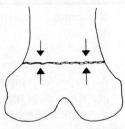

4. portion of metaphysis, growth plate & epiphysis

5. crushing of growth plate

Fig. 17.11. Growth plate fractures

★★★ Type 3 and type 4 fractures are seen occasionally and behave similarly to oblique condyle fractures in the adult (Fig. 17.11). They should undergo open reduction in order to obtain an anatomical position.

**** Type 5 crushing injuries to the growth plate of the femur are seen in children after road traffic accidents or falls from a height (Fig. 17.11). Unfortunately it is frequently impossible to diagnose them from X-rays.

These children may well present some years later with a short leg or a knee deformity. In any case treatment in the acute stage is of little avail.

Fractures involving the upper articular surface of the tibia
*** Depressed fractures of the upper tibia
*** Split fractures of the upper tibia
**** Split and depressed fractures of the upper tibia
*** Avulsion fractures of the upper tibia

*** *Depressed fractures of the upper tibia* (Fig. 17.12a)
The articular surface of the upper end of the tibia consists of a plateau of thin cortical bone, beneath which are arcades of cancellous bone. Abduction or adduction injuries of the knee in the middle aged or the elderly will result in the femoral shaft being forced into the tibial plateau. This causes a depressed fracture of the cortical plateau and compression of the under-lying trabeculae of cancellous bone. It is difficult to obtain and maintain an anatomical reduction of these fractures. There may be associated ligament damage.

An abduction force causes a depression of the lateral tibial condyle. This is seen frequently in pedestrians struck by a car. It is known as a 'bumper fracture'. There may be associated rupture of the medial ligament.

An adduction force will cause a depression fracture of the

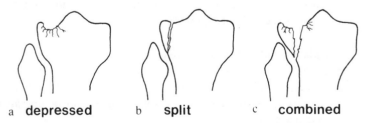

a **depressed**   b **split**   c **combined**

Fig. 17.12.   Fracture of the tibial condyles

medial tibial condyle. This lesion may be associated with rupture of the lateral ligament.

The patient with a depressed fracture of the upper tibia presents with a bruised painful knee and a haemarthrosis. If the depression is severe there may be observable varus or valgus deformity of the knee. Ideally these fractures should be reduced anatomically as the knee is a weight-bearing joint. In practice this is only attempted if there is severe degree of depression or the knee is unstable or both.

Complications
Knee stiffness is common and these patients should be mobilised as soon as practical and encouraged to do non-weight-bearing exercises.

Malunion results from healing of the depressed fracture. A varus or valgus deformity results. This deformity is more marked if there is any residual ligament laxity.

Degenerative changes in the knee are liable to occur. These may cause little in the way of symptoms for many years. As the patient is usually elderly to start with they may never become a problem requiring treatment.

** *Fractures with minimal depression* should have the haemarthrosis aspirated. A plaster cylinder is then applied and retained for three weeks — the patient uses crutches non-weight-bearing. Following this the plaster is bivalved and the knee mobilised with non weight-bearing exercises from the plaster back slab.

*** *Fractures with considerable depression or instability* should undergo operation. The fracture can be elevated and held in position by packing bone chips beneath it. If the medial ligament is disrupted it can be repaired at the same time. A plaster back slab is applied and skeletal traction set up. After a week active exercises are started. The patient must remain non-weight bearing for at least eight weeks.

Split fractures of the upper tibia
*** *Split fractures of the tibial condyle* (Fig. 17.12b). These occur in younger patients. The tibial plateau is split rather than depressed. If the fracture is displaced it should be operated on and fixed with a bolt.

**** *Split fractures of the tibial condyle with depression* (Fig. 17.12c). These occur occasionally and are a difficult problem. Not only is the tibial plateau depressed but a portion is split away. The only way the fracture can be held reduced is by open reduction and fixation with a bolt. The articular surface has to be elevated and supported by cancellous bone grafts. Even so an inadequate reduction often results.

Avulsion fractures
Tibial spine fractures
Posterior marginal fractures

These fractures usually represent avulsion fractures of ligament attachments. Their treatment is but part of the treatment of ligament injuries. A good result can be obtained from open reduction and fixation of the bone fragments.

*** *A fracture of the tibial spine* represents an avulsion of the anterior cruciate ligament attachment (Fig. 17.6). It occurs mainly in children and adolescents as a result of bicycle or sports injuries. The patient has a swollen knee and a haemarthrosis.

If the fragment is undisplaced the knee should be aspirated and immobilised in a plaster cylinder for a few weeks. If the fragment is significantly displaced it is best to operate and fix the fragment with pins.

*** *A posterior marginal fracture* represents a rupture of the posterior cruciate ligament (Fig. 17.5). It is most frequently seen as a dashboard injury following road traffic accidents. An untreated posterior cruciate ligament injury is a very serious disability. The lesion should be operated on if at all possible and the fragment reduced and the posterior capsule and posterior cruciate repaired.

18 Injuries of the Tibia and Fibula

*** Fractures of the middle and lower thirds of the tibia and fibula
** Isolated fractures of the tibia
** Spiral fractures of the tibia and fibula
*** Fractures of the upper third of the tibia and fibula
**** Fractures of the lower end of the tibia
* Isolated fractures of the fibula
** Fractures of the tibia and fibula in children
*** Dislocations of the superior tibiofibular joint

The tibia is superficial throughout its length. Fractures of the tibia are frequently complicated by skin wounds and become compound fractures.

As the tibia is superficial it is fatally easy to do an operation and plate the fracture. Unfortunately even though the skin is overtly intact it may be covertly damaged. Skin sloughing and infection occur only too frequently after such an operation.

A torsional stress produces a spiral fracture of the tibia. This is a low energy fracture such as occurs frequently after skiing accidents. There is relatively little soft tissue damage.

Direct violence and bending forces produce high energy fractures with a relatively severe damage to skin and soft tissue. The bone fragments are more severely involved and a greater portion of bone loses its blood supply. Delayed union and non-union of these types of fractures occur frequently.

The popliteal artery bifurcates into anterior and posterior tibial arteries at the upper end of the interosseous membrane. The artery is tethered at this site and liable to damage from a displaced fracture of the upper third of the tibia.

The lower leg in enclosed in deep fascia. This encloses four well-defined and localised fascial compartments. These are (see Fig. 1.19):

anterior tibial compartment;
peroneal compartment (laterally);
superficial posterior compartment;
deep posterior compartment.

168

These compartments can remain intact after fractures of the tibia. The deep muscles are damaged and bleed causing an increase in pressure in the closed compartment. Venous stasis and later insufficiency of arterial blood supply results. Eventually the muscle in the compartment dies and the necrotic mass becomes replaced by fibrous tissue — a contracture results.

The patient complains of severe pain and has a very swollen leg. There is associated tingling and paraesthesiae. However, the peripheral pulses may be present until a late stage — the capillary return and skin colour over the foot may remain normal.

If this condition is suspected an operation known as a fasciotomy should be performed to release the affected compartments.

*** Fractures of the middle and lower thirds of the shafts of the tibia and fibula

These transverse, oblique or comminuted fractures are mainly high energy fractures resulting from considerable violence (Fig. 18.1). They are often associated with other general injuries. They may be associated with a fracture of the ipsilateral femur.

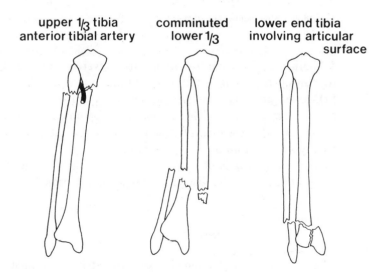

Fig. 18.1. Fractures of the tibia

Chapter 18

Complications

1 Compound fracture. These are frequently compound injuries. Often the skin is intact but badly contused. Such skin damage is seen with crushing or degloving injuries.

2 Malunion. This consists of angulation after imperfect reduction. The alignment of the fracture must be almost perfect in the A-P view. An angulation of ten degrees is allowable in the lateral view.

3 A rotational deformity also occurs. The mid-inguinal point, patella, and great toe should be in a straight line (Fig. 18.2).

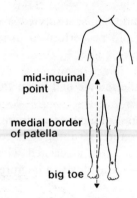

Fig. 18.2. Alignment of the tibia

4 Shortening is liable to occur after severely comminuted fractures. Shortening within one centimetre is acceptable.

5 Delayed union and non-union. These occur frequently after high energy fractures. The normal time for union is thirteen weeks but the fracture of any particular patient may take twenty weeks to unite.

After this length of time a grafting operation using cancellous bone from the iliac crest should be performed.

Management

First aid

These fractures can be immobilised adequately in an inflatable splint. Failing this a right angled splint can be used. Other severe injuries may cause hypovolaemic shock which requires emergency treatment.

Initial treatment

This involves manipulative reduction and immobilisation in a long leg plaster. A compound fracture should be operated on at this early stage. These fractures are often unstable and difficult to immobilise in plaster. A pin through the calcaneum can steady the distal fragment so that it can be incorporated in plaster. After immobilisation in the long leg plaster, the plaster and the underlying padding should be split throughout its length so that it can be easily loosened if there is excessive swelling.

If the fracture cannot be reduced and maintained in plaster a pin should be inserted in the calcaneum and traction applied (Fig. 18.3). When the patient's condition has stabilised the fracture is plated. If the fracture is comminuted a cancellous graft can be applied at the same time.

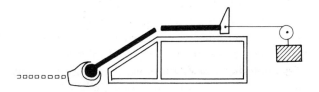

Fig. 18.3. Calcaneus traction

If there is extensive skin damage or skin loss the fractured tibia is maintained in some sort of external fixation apparatus. This can provide rigid fixation. Wound debridement and skin grafts can then be performed without disturbing the fracture (Fig. 18.4).

Definitive treatment

The safest method of treating fractures of the tibia and fibula is by using an above-knee plaster until union occurs. When the fracture is fairly stable, a patella bearing plaster or a plastic cast brace, can be applied and weight bearing and knee mobilisation commenced.

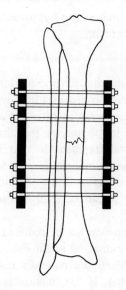

Fig. 18.4. External fixateur

Operation on a fractured tibia is indicated for:
1 Compound injuries − internal fixation is not used in association on account of the dangers of infection.
2 Double fracture of the tibia. These are probably best controlled by fixation with an intramedullary nail.
3 Fixation of fractures of femur and tibia on the same side.
4 Unstable fractures which cannot be stabilised by closed means.
5 A below-knee amputation may be necessary for a badly damaged limb.

** **Isolated fractures of the tibia**
These are fairly common direct violence injuries. They may result from soccer injuries after a direct kick on the skin.

The fractures are frequently undisplaced. If they are displaced reduction may be difficult by closed means as the intact fibula acts as a splint.

Isolated fractures of the tibia can be complicated by a closed compartment syndrome. It is wise to admit these patients to hospital for twenty-four hours to exclude this complication.

The fractures can be immobilised in an above-knee plaster for thirteen weeks until union. A patella bearing plaster or a plastic cast brace can be applied after four weeks to permit knee movements.

A displaced fracture may be difficult to reduce and open reduction and plating may be indicated.

** Spiral fractures of the tibia and fibula

These fractures result from torsional violence as occurs from the majority of skiing injuries.

The patient has an obvious fracture clinically. The lower leg lies in external rotation if the fracture is displaced.

Undisplaced fractures may be treated in an above-knee plaster.

Displaced fractures require reduction under general anaesthetic and an above-knee plaster is applied. The patient should be kept in hospital for two or three days before going home.

He may then be mobilised non-weight-bearing on crutches for four weeks — following which he can weight bear in plaster. Union usually takes three months.

Spiral fractures unite readily. The main complication is malunion from inadequate reduction.

*** Fractures of the upper third of the tibia and fibula

These are not so common but can represent severe injuries. The popliteal artery can be damaged by displaced fractures in the region of its bifurcation (Fig. 18.1).

The treatment is similar to other fractures of the tibia. The fractures can usually be reduced adequately by manipulation and are reasonably stable in plaster.

**** Fractures of the lower end of the tibia

These fractures may have an extension into the ankle joint. They are liable to be complicated by ankle stiffness (Fig. 18.1).

The fragments may be difficult to control by closed means and open reduction and fixation with plate and screws is often necessary.

173

* **Isolated fractures of the fibula**

These occur frequently. However, an injury of the ankle below the lesion must be excluded.

A fracture of the neck of the fibula may be associated with a peroneal nerve injury producing a foot drop.

They can be treated by a supporting bandage, local applications and exercises. Many patients are more comfortable in a below-knee walking plaster for three weeks.

** **Fractures of the tibia and fibula in children**

These fractures can almost always be managed conservatively. They unite readily. Children have an excellent capacity for remodelling and malunion is only a problem if rotation is not adequately corrected.

Fractures of the upper third of the tibia can be associated with damage to the growth plate. Shortening and deformity can result.

*** **Dislocation of the superior tibiofibular joint**

These follow severe falls or road traffic accidents. They may be associated with displaced fractures of the tibia or displaced fractures of the ankle.

The patient with an isolated injury complains of a feeling of weakness and discomfort in the knee and swelling of the head of the fibula.

On examination there is a prominence of the head of the fibula and careful perusal of X-rays confirms diagnosis.

The lesion is usually reducible by manipulation under general anaesthetic. The reduction is usually stable.

19 Injuries of the Ankle

   * Ankle sprains
  ** Lateral ligament rupture
  ** Undisplaced fracture of medial or lateral malleolus
 *** Displaced ankle fractures — Potts' fractures
 *** Osteochondral fractures
 *** Rupture of tendo achilles

Injuries to the ankle joint involve ligaments as well as bone.
The X-ray picture may not reveal the true extent of the lesion.
An undisplaced and seemingly benign ankle fracture may have
associated major ligament damage — such a lesion is unstable.

A displaced fracture of the bones about the ankle represents
a subluxation of the ankle joint. Such a displaced fracture-
subluxation is generally called a Potts' fracture. Displaced
fractures of the ankle require anatomical reduction otherwise
symptomatic degenerative changes are inevitable.

The lower end of the tibia and the lateral malleolus of the
fibula are firmly held together by an interosseous ligament.
They form a mortice for the talus. If the interosseous ligament
is disrupted the fibula tends to float away from the tibia
causing a diastasis of the ankle joint (Fig. 19.1). If the ankle is
allowed to heal with a diastasis unreduced the joint is made
incongrous and degenerative changes are inevitable.

Lateral stability of the ankle depends on the anterior talofibular ligament as well as the calcaneofibular ligament. An
inversion force frequently causes damage to the anterior talofibular ligament and a sprained ankle results. A more serious
injury also causes damage to the calcaneofibular ligament,
producing the syndrome of rupture of the lateral ligaments of
the ankle (Fig. 19.2).

Posteriorly the ankle joint is controlled by the posterior
talofibular and the posterior tibiofibular ligament. The posterior
tibiofibular ligament is attached to the prominence on the
posterior margin of the lower end of the tibia. This prominence

175

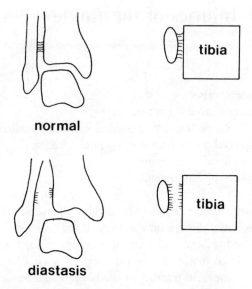

normal

diastasis

Fig. 19.1. Interosseous ligament

is sometimes known as the posterior malleolus of the tibia (or third malleolus) (Fig. 19.3).

The posterior tibiofibular ligament may be detached in a type of injury due to an external rotation force acting on the ankle. The foot is plantar flexed and fixed and the body and lower leg moves forwards. The foot is forced backwards relative to the lower leg. The posterior malleolus is fractured and may take with it a considerable portion of the articular surface of the tibia (Fig. 19.3).

The medial side of the ankle is controlled by the strong deltoid ligament (Fig. 19.4). This can be damaged by abduction or external rotation forces. If the ligament is ruptured the diagnosis depends on clinical examination and inference from the position of the bones on X-ray. Frequently the medial malleolus is avulsed instead of the ligament being ruptured (Fig. 19.4). Ankle fractures can be produced by:

1 External rotation forces:
   with the foot prone (dorsiflexed and everted);
   with the foot supine (plantar flexed and inverted).
2 Abduction forces.

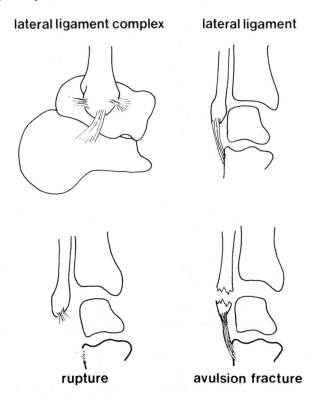

lateral ligament complex   **lateral ligament**

rupture   **avulsion fracture**

Fig. 19.2. Lateral side injuries

3 Adduction forces.

4 Vertical compression forces.

On dorsiflexing the foot the talus also twists in the ankle mortice so that the lateral malleolus articulates with the anterior portion of the facet on the lateral side of the talus. When the foot is plantar flexed it articulates with the posterior portion of the facet (Fig. 19.5).

An external rotation force applied to the ankle with the foot in dorsiflexion causes either a rupture of the medial ligament or an avulsion of the medial malleolus. It will also tend to disrupt the interosseous ligament and fracture the lateral malleolus (Fig. 19.6).

There is a particular injury which causes rupture of both medial and interosseous ligaments and also causes an oblique

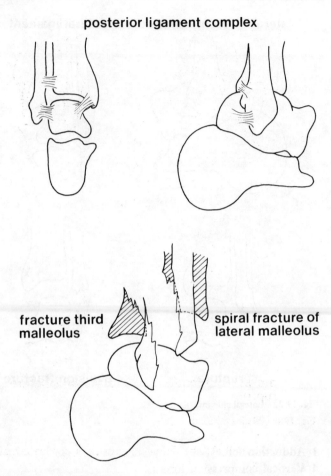

posterior ligament complex

fracture third malleolus

spiral fracture of lateral malleolus

Fig. 19.3. Posterior injuries

fracture of the lateral malleolus just above the joint line. This lesion is easily reduced by splintage and may appear on X-ray as an undisplaced fracture (Fig. 19.6). If inadequately treated the position can be lost in plaster and the ankle can heal with an unreduced diastasis.

An external rotation force applied with the foot in plantar flexion will tend to twist the lateral malleolus on the rest of the fibula causing a spiral fracture. The interosseous ligament remains intact (Fig. 19.7). If the foot is forced backwards (or the body and rest of the limb forwards), the posterior structure

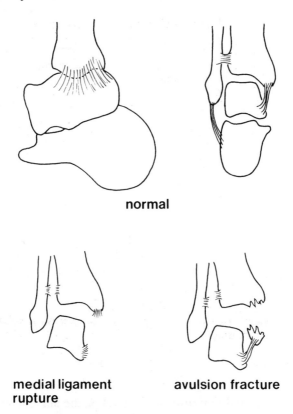

normal

**medial ligament
rupture**

avulsion fracture

Fig. 19.4. Medial ligament

of the ankle will also be damaged causing a posterior malleolar fracture (Fig. 19.3).

Abduction violence tends to avulse the medial malleolus rather than rupture the medial ligament. The lateral malleolus

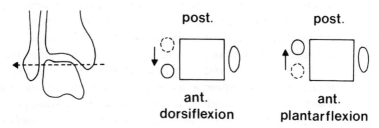

post.

post.

**ant.
dorsiflexion**

**ant.
plantarflexion**

Fig. 19.5. Lateral malleolus and talus

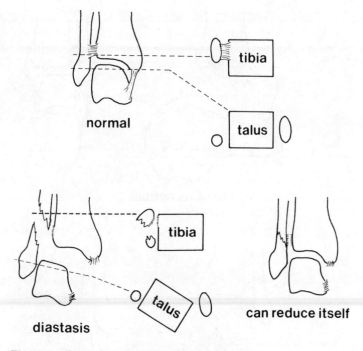

Fig. 19.6. External rotation of dorsiflexed ankle

is fractured outwards at the level of the ankle joint — this is known as a shear fracture (Fig. 19.8).

Abduction violence can also cause a more severe injury tearing the interosseous ligament and fracturing the fibula above it. The X-ray is very similar to that produced by an external rotation in dorsiflexion injury (Fig. 19.8). On occasions the talus is interposed between the tibia and fibula producing a Dupuytren's fracture dislocation.

Adduction force will cause the lateral ligament complex to rupture or a fracture of the lateral malleolus. In more severe injuries there is also a fracture of the medial malleolus, part of the articular surface of this fracture is comminuted (Fig. 19.9).

A vertical compression force can produce a variety of injuries from a minor anterior marginal fracture to a comminuted fracture-subluxation which damages the joint irretrievably.

The evaluation of displacement of an ankle fracture depends on good quality X-rays.

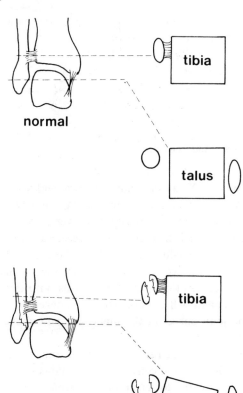

Fig. 19.7. External rotation of plantarflexed ankle

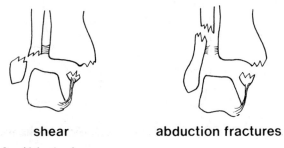

shear   abduction fractures

Fig. 19.8. Abduction fractures

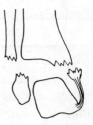

Fig. 19.9. Adduction fracture

An A-P X-ray of a normal ankle will show the joint space between the talus and the medial malleolus and the joint space between the talus and the lower end of the tibia as being even and equal throughout. There is a concavity of the upper border of the talus which matches precisely the convexity of the lower surface of the tibia. (In the normal A-P there is some overlap of the lateral malleolus onto the talus.) A slight displacement will be revealed as an unevenness and an inequality of the joint space on the inner side and above the talus (Fig. 19.10).

The lateral X-ray of a normal ankle will show an even joint space and the convexity of the talus matches precisely the concavity of the lower end of the tibia.

It is essential that these X-rays are properly centred and are true A-P and lateral views.

* *An ankle sprain* results from an inversion force. The common lesion is damage of the anterior talofibular ligament. The

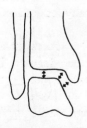
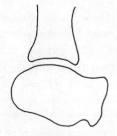

A –P normal x-ray   **lateral**

Fig. 19.10. Normal X-ray of ankle

patient complains of bruising and swelling of the outer side of the ankle.

An ankle sprain can be treated simply by supportive strapping and early weight bearing exercises.

** *A rupture of the lateral ligament* of the ankle involves disruption of the calcaneofibular ligament as well as the anterior talofibular ligament. The lesion is unstable. If the patient is allowed unrestricted exercise healing will be incomplete and recurrent laxity of the lateral ligament results.

These patients have similar but more severe physical signs and negative X-ray findings. If a lateral ligament rupture is suspected the limb can be immobilised in a below-knee walking plaster for four weeks.

The diagnosis can be made certain by doing stress X-rays under an anaesthetic or by performing arthrograms. These must be performed if there is any question of operating on the ankle.

** *Undisplaced fractures of the ankle* are best treated by immobilisation in a below-knee plaster for six weeks. In the acute phase a below-knee plaster slab is used and the patient elevates the limb until swelling subsides. Later a complete below-knee walking plaster is applied.

An undisplaced fracture of the lateral malleolus above the joint line must be treated with caution. There may be an associated rupture of both medial and interosseous ligaments. As the swelling subsides and the plaster works loose the fracture will tend to become displaced. It is wise to check the position of these fractures by X-ray through the plaster.

*** *Potts' fractures* (fracture dislocations of the ankle)
These fractures must be anatomically reduced and the reduction must be maintained.

Manipulative reduction may be successful and plaster immobilisation for eight weeks may be adequate. However, these fractures require careful monitoring and repeat X-rays in the plaster after two weeks, should be taken to make sure the position is maintained. After four weeks the plaster can be changed for weight bearing plaster and a further X-ray taken.

Certain lesions usually require open reduction and fixation:
1 A displaced fracture of the medial malleolus is often difficult

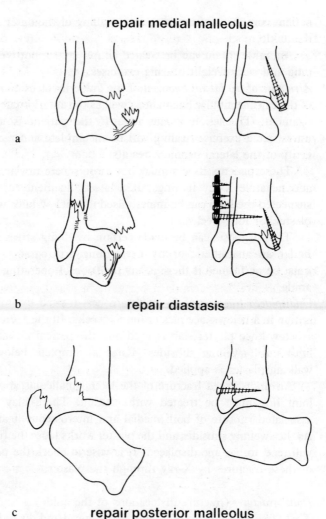

repair medial malleolus

a

b

repair diastasis

c

repair posterior malleolus

Fig. 19.11. Operations for ankle fractures

to reduce anatomically by manipulation. A fold of periosteum is liable to be caught between the bone fragments. At operation this fold of periosteum is extricated and the fragment fixed with a screw (Fig. 19.11a).

2 A diastasis is often difficult to manage in plaster. As swelling resolves and the plaster becomes loose the fibula tends to float away from the tibia.

The fracture of the fibula can be reduced at operation and fixed with plate and screws. The lower-most screw can be passed across into the tibia along the line of the interosseous ligament — it will hold the diastasis reduced (Fig. 19.11b). In due course the plate and screws will have to be removed as continual fretting will cause the diastasis screw to break.

3 A large posterior fragment requires accurate reduction to restore the articular surface of the lower end of the tibia. This very frequently necessitates open reduction (Fig. 19.11c).

4 Any fracture which cannot be adequately reduced by closed means should undergo open reduction. Any fracture which becomes displaced again after closed reduction should have an operation.

*** *Osteochondral fractures* occur occasionally from the upper surface of the talus. They may be associated with other ankle fractures. Osteochondral fractures do not usually heal and the fragment remains loose causing pain and instability. They are best removed at arthrotomy.

*** *Rupture of the tendo achilles*
The tendo achilles becomes degenerate with age. A rupture is liable to occur through this degenerate portion. At operation,

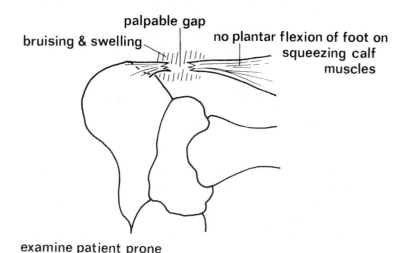

examine patient prone

Fig. 19.12. Tests for ruptured tendo achilles

the tendon appears as a mass of degenerate fibrous tissue with clot and even calcification interposed between the fibres. The patient complains of sudden pain in the back of the heel (as though being hit). It usually occurs whilst running or during sporting activity of some sort. On examination, the back of the lower leg is swollen. There may be a palpable gap in the tendo achilles. The 'squeeze test' may be positive. The patient lies prone with the foot just over the edge of the examination couch. Squeezing of the gastrocnemius−soleus complex in the normal leg will cause the foot to plantar flex. If the tendo achilles is ruptured, then there will be no such plantar flexion (Fig. 19.12).

The best results are obtained by performing an open operation. At operation, the clot and degenerative tissue is cleaned out and the ends of the tendon are approximated and sutured. The leg must be maintained in a below-knee plaster with the foot plantar flexed for about seven or eight weeks. Patients frequently present late with this lesion. In such cases, it is permissible to offer them no definite treatment as the results of active treatment at this stage are not so satisfactory, and the residual disability may not be great.

20 Foot Injuries

★★ The crushed foot
★★★ Dislocations of the foot
★★ Fractures of the talus
★★★ Fractures of the calcaneum
 ★ Flake fractures of the tarsus
★★ Fractures of the metatarsals
 ★ Fractures of the phalanges

★★ The crushed foot
Most serious foot injuries result from direct violence, causing
some degree of crushing of the soft tissues. These injuries
cause considerable bruising, swelling and pain. The overlying
skin may be damaged by lacerations and abrasions.

Fractures which appear trivial on X-ray may be accompanied
by considerable pain and swelling from soft tissue damage. The
patient's convalescence is necessarily prolonged. Very occasionally the swelling is such that operative decompression of
the foot is necessary to release the pent-up haematoma.

Treatment of the fracture involves treatment of the swollen
foot. This includes rest, elevation and local applications of ice.
This treatment is often best accomplished in hospital.

Following such an injury the patient will complain of pain
and stiffness and recurrent swelling in the foot for a considerable period of time. Residual symptoms of tingling and hyperaesthesia may persist for months.

★★★ Dislocations of the foot
There are many joints in the foot and dislocations have been
described involving every one of them. They are not common
but are often associated with complications and difficulties in
management. Lesions to be considered:
Total dislocation of the talus
Fracture dislocation of the body of the talus
Subtalar dislocation
Tarsometatarsal fracture dislocation

Dislocation of the metatarsophalangeal or the interphalangeal joints of the toes

**** *Total dislocation of the talus* is rare. It is an injury which used to be seen in aviators who crashed (and survived). The talus is extruded from the ankle mortice and comes to rest on the anterior aspect of the foot and ankle. The lesion is often compound.

The dislocation is reduced, if necessary by open operation. Avascular necrosis of the talus is inevitable.

**** *Fracture dislocation of the body of the talus* is now more common. This results from a severe injury, usually a car or motorcycle accident. The patient frequently has severe multiple injuries which demand urgent attention.

The talus fractures at its neck, and the body (which articulates at the ankle joint) is extruded posteromedially (Fig. 20.1). There are usually associated fractures of the ankle. The dislocated portion impinges on the posterior tibial nerve and vessels

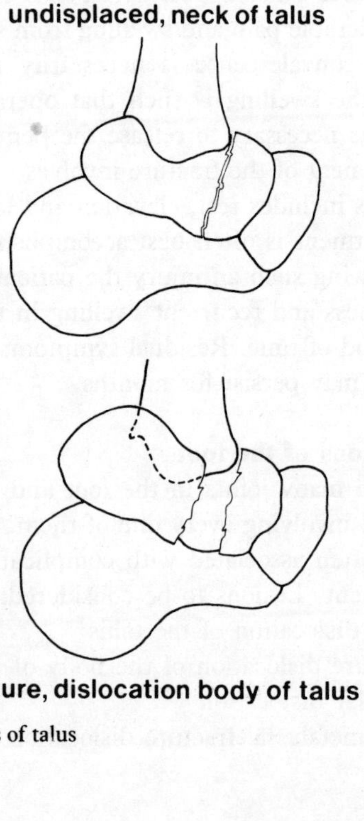

undisplaced, neck of talus

fracture, dislocation body of talus

Fig. 20.1. Fractures of talus

and also presses on the overlying skin. The viability of the whole foot is compromised.

The lesion should be reduced as soon as possible — open reduction is usually necessary.

Avascular necrosis of the talus is a frequent late complication.

** *Subtalar dislocation* occurs occasionally as a result of an inversion injury. The patient has a painful, swollen and obviously deformed foot.

The dislocation requires reduction as soon as possible by manipulation under general anaesthetic. Open reduction is occasionally required if closed reduction is blocked by small bone fragments.

The late complication of subtalar dislocation is stiffness of the subtalar joint — residual pain is not usually a problem and further treatment should not be necessary. Avascular necrosis of the talus is not a complication.

*** *Tarsometatarsal fracture dislocation* occurs occasionally after motorcycle accidents. The metatarsals are dislocated laterally — the base of the second metatarsal is usually fractured (see Fig. 20.3). Sometimes the first metatarsal is dislocated medially.

This lesion is easily reduced but the reduction is unstable. It is best to perform an open reduction fixing it with pins. Decompression of the foot can be performed at the same time.

If the lesion is not reduced the patient is left with an ugly stiff flat foot due to the residual abduction deformity of the forefoot.

** *Dislocations of the metatarsophalangeal and interphalangeal joints of the toes.* These are usually minor injuries and can be reduced simply by manipulation. The reduction is usually stable and can be maintained by strapping to an adjacent toe.

Fractures of the talus

The talus has blood supply from various sources. However, its proximal portion (the body) is largely articular. If it is dislocated it will lose its blood supply and is liable later to develop avascular necrosis.

Avascular necrosis always occurs after a total dislocation and frequently after a fracture dislocation of the body. It only rarely occurs after a fracture of the neck without dislocation.

The body of the talus collapses and becomes dense on X-ray after avascular necrosis — degenerative changes occur in both ankle and subtalar joints. The patient has an incapacitatingly painful and stiff ankle and foot. This condition is usually treated by arthrodesis of both ankle and subtalar joints — a pantalar arthrodesis — and the patient is left with a very significant disability.

Injuries of the talus are varied:

total dislocation (p. 188)

fracture dislocation of the body of the talus (p. 188)

subtalar dislocation (p.189)

fracture of the neck of the talus

flake fractures of the talus (p. 192)

** *Fractures of the neck of the talus* are seen occasionally after severe injuries such as falls from a height and road traffic accidents. There are often other severe injuries (Fig. 20.1).

The patient has a painful, swollen and bruised foot. He should be admitted to hospital. The foot is supported in a well padded below-knee plaster slab and the foot elevated.

After the swelling has resolved a full below-knee plaster can be applied and the patient remains non-weight-bearing for six weeks after injury. A walking plaster can then be used for a further three weeks.

Fractures of the calcaneum

The calcaneus is made of cancellous bone. The mid and anterior portions of the superior aspect articulate with the talus at the subtalar joint.

The majority of fractures of the calcaneum result from falls from a height. The fractures are often crush fractures with the trabeculae compressed together. The articular surface of the subtalar joint is often damaged and stiffness and degenerative changes are late complications.

Falls from a height may produce other injuries. The other foot and heel should be carefully examined as calcaneus fractures are often bilateral. The back should also be carefully examined and X-rayed to exclude a crush fracture in the dorsi-lumbar region.

Fractures of the calcaneum can be missed. The patient may complain of pain in the ankle and that region is examined and

Foot Injuries

X-rayed. It is wise to examine all patients complaining of ankle injuries from behind. Only in this way can some calcaneus fractures and ruptures of the tendo achilles be detected. It is also wise to include a view of the calcaneum when X-raying the ankle.

Patients present with several kinds of fractures of the calcaneum:

avulsion fractures of the insertion of the tendo achilles (fractures of the sustentaculum tali)
oblique fractures not involving the subtalar joint
crush fractures involving the subtalar joint
flake fractures of the calcaneum (p. 192)

*** *Avulsion fractures of the insertion of the tendo achilles* occur only occasionally. The fracture requires open reduction and internal fixation. Following this the foot and ankle must be immobilised in plaster with the foot in plantar flexion.

** *Oblique fractures not involving the subtalar joint* are frequently difficult to see on X-ray (Fig. 20.2). An axial view of the calcaneum may be necessary.

This is not a severe injury and there may be little bruising and swelling. The patient can be immobilised in a well padded below-knee plaster slab and the foot elevated. When the swelling has subsided a below-knee walking plaster can be applied and retained until four weeks from fracture.

Even so considerable mobilising exercises may be necessary before the patient is fit to return to work.

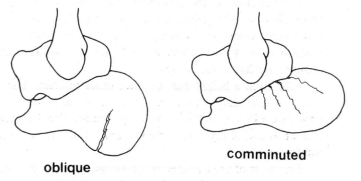

oblique

comminuted

Fig. 20.2. Fractures of calcaneum

*** *Crush fractures involving the subtalar joint* (Fig. 20.2)

These represent a severe injury to the foot. They usually result from falls from a height — the patient landing on his heels. He has considerable bruising and swelling and a very painful foot. There may be associated injuries. The other foot and the lumbar spine should be carefully examined.

Patients with this injury should be admitted to hospital and treated with bed rest and elevation of the foot. Active exercises are encouraged. When the swelling has resolved a below-knee plaster is applied and the patient immobilised non-weight-bearing with crutches. Weight bearing in plaster is permitted after five or six weeks.

Convalescence is prolonged. The patient may complain of pain and stiffness in the subtalar joint for months. A subtalar or triple arthrodesis may be necessary.

Because of this prolonged convalescence operative treatment is sometimes recommended. Open reduction and elevation of the fragments by a bone graft is described. Early triple arthrodesis has been recommended. Unfortunately the results of these procedures are uncertain.

Flake fractures of the tarsus

These occur frequently after minor torsional injuries to the foot. They probably represent avulsion of ligament attachments. Flake fractures are seen arising from the talus, the calcaneum and the cuboid.

These patients can be treated symptomatically with strapping and active exercises. If the patient will not tolerate this a below-knee walking plaster can be used for some three weeks.

Fractures of the metatarsals
** Transverse or comminuted fractures
* Oblique fractures
* Fractures through the base of the fifth metacarpal
** Stress fractures
*** Tarsometatarsal fracture dislocations (p. 189)

Fractures of the metatarsals can occur from minor torsional injuries. Usually oblique fractures or fractures of the neck arise in this manner. They require simple treatment.

Transverse or comminuted fractures result from direct violence and crushing injuries. Treatment of these patients involves management of the severely damaged soft tissues.

** *Transverse or comminuted fractures* of the metatarsals usually indicate crushing injury with significant damage to skin and soft tissues.

These fractures can be reduced (if necessary) by manipulation under general anaesthetic and the foot immobilised in a well padded below-knee plaster. The patient should be admitted to hospital and the foot elevated until the swelling subsides. Following this is a below-knee walking plaster can be applied and continued until four weeks from injury.

Exercises and physiotherapy to reduce swelling are then usually necessary and the convalescence from work may last for some two or three months.

If there is severe displacement of the fractures the opportunity should be taken to operate and perform a decompression of the foot at the same time as the open reduction.

* *Oblique fractures of metatarsals* occur frequently from torsional injuries. These patients can be treated with a below-knee plaster

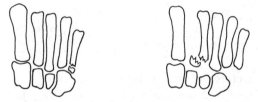

a

5th metatarsal base   metarsotarsal dislocation

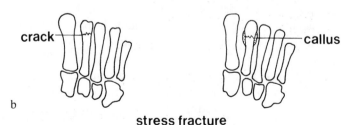

crack   callus

b

stress fracture

Fig. 20.3.   Fractures of metatarsals

slab and elevation of the foot at home. Following this the foot can be mobilized with only strapping as support.

* *Fractures of the base of the fifth metatarsal* are very common as a result of a twisting injury to the foot (Fig. 20.3a). The lesion may represent an avulsion of the attachment of peroneus brevis.

   These patients can be treated symptomatically with strapping and active exercises. Some people require immobilisation in a below-knee plaster for three weeks.

   Occasionally a patient will have persisting discomfort from an ununited fragment. These symptoms will resolve in due course.

** *Stress fractures of the metatarsal necks* (Fig. 20.3b)
Usually the second metatarsal is involved. This lesion occurs after a long walk or route march — when the patient is unaccustomed to such exercise. It used to be seen in army recruits.

   The patient will complain of severe metatarsal pain — there may be only slight swelling. An X-ray will show no lesion or only a very ill defined crack. An X-ray taken some weeks later will show a cloud of healing callus. A bone scan is a much more sensitive diagnostic indicator of a stress fracture.

   The patient therefore is best diagnosed on the history and treated with rest in a below-knee plaster for three weeks — symptoms will then resolve.

Fractures of the phalanges of the toes
These fractures can result from crushing injuries or from torsional injuries.

** Crushing injuries of the toes require treatment for the soft tissue damage. The limb can then be immobilised in a below-knee plaster slab with a toe platform. Elevation is usually adequate if the patient rests at home in bed. The fractures are usually united by the time the soft tissues are healed.

   Convalescence from work may well be six or eight weeks.

* Torsional injuries can usually be managed by strapping to an adjacent toe. Sometimes the fractures is displaced sufficiently to warrant manipulative reduction. Strapping is usually adequate to hold the position.

Further Reading

CHARNLEY J. (1970) *Closed Treatment of Common Fractures* (2nd edn), Churchill Livingstone, Edinburgh.

CRAWFORD-ADAMS J. (1984) *Outline of Fractures* (8th edn), Churchill Livingstone, Edinburgh.

EDMONSON A.S. & CRENSHAW A.H. (1980) *Campbell's Operative Orthopaedics* (5th edn), Mosby, St Louis.

MULLER M.E., ALLGOWER M. & WILLENEGGER H. (1979) *Manual of Internal Fixation* (2nd edn), Springer-Verlag, Berlin.

RANG M. (1982) *Children's Fractures* (2nd edn), Lippincott, Philadelphia.

ROCKWOOD C.A. & GREEN D.P. (Eds) (1984) *Fractures* (2nd edn) (3 vols), Lippincott, Philadelphia.

WILSON J.N. (Ed.) (1983) *Watson—Jones Fractures and Joint Injuries* (6th edn), Churchill Livingstone, Edinburgh.

Sensation to foot
   sciatic
     lat & medial plantar
     deep peroneal
     superficial "
     saphenous
     sural
     tibial

Index

Index

Index

Index

Index

Index

Index